SENTENCED TO SCIENCE

THE PENNSYLVANIA STATE UNIVERSITY PRESS
UNIVERSITY PARK, PENNSYLVANIA

SENTENCED TO SCIENCE

ONE BLACK MAN'S STORY OF IMPRISONMENT IN AMERICA

ALLEN M. HORNBLUM

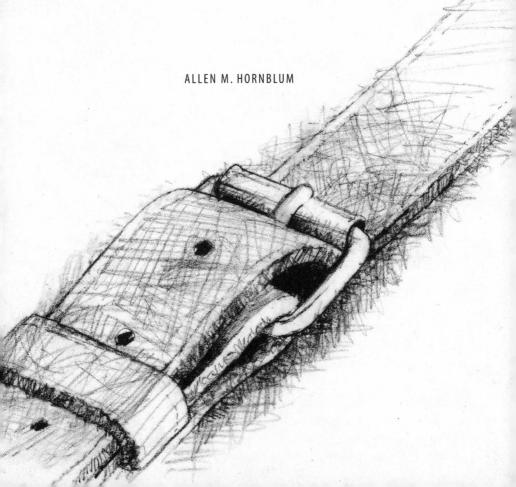

Library of Congress
Cataloging-in-Publication Data

Hornblum, Allen M.
Sentenced to Science : one black man's story of
imprisonment in America /
Allen M. Hornblum
P.   cm.
Includes bibliographical references and index.
ISBN 978-0-271-03336-5 (cloth : alk. paper)
1. Human experimentation in medicine—
Pennsylvania—Philadelphia.
2. Anthony, Edward, 1943–.
3. Prisoners—Pennsylvania—Philadelphia—Anecdotes.
4. Holmesburg Prison.
I. Title.

[DNLM: 1. Anthony, Edward, 1943–. 2. Holmesburg
Prison. 3. Human Experimentation—Philadelphia—
Personal Narratives. 4. African Americans—
Philadelphia—Personal Narratives. 5. Prisoners—
Philadelphia—Personal Narratives. 6. Prisons—
Philadelphia. W 20.55.H9 H814s 2007]

R853.H8H67 2007
615.5072'40974811—dc22
2007017451

The Pennsylvania State University Press
is a member of the Association of
American University Presses.

It is the policy of The Pennsylvania State University
Press to use acid-free paper. This book is printed on
Natures Natural, containing 50% post-consumer
waste, and meets the minimum requirements of
American National Standard for Information
Sciences—Permanence of Paper for Printed Library
Material, ANSI Z39.48–1992.

CONTENTS

To those physicians and researchers who
chose not to use vulnerable,
institutionalized populations as test subjects
for their experiments.

The degree of civilization in a society can be
judged by entering its prisons.

—FYODOR DOSTOEVSKY

ACKNOWLEDGMENTS

The publication of *Acres of Skin* during the summer of 1998 attracted remarkable media interest, both here and abroad. The television, radio, and newsprint coverage not only helped illuminate a dark chapter in American medical history but also signaled a clarion call for former Holmesburg Prison test subjects—at long last they would learn the truth about the strange medical experiments in which they had once participated.

Dozens, then scores, of former Holmesburg prisoners began showing up at various neighborhood meetings. Renewing old acquaintances and making new ones, the men and women—mostly African American and in their sixties and seventies now—had two things in common: they had once been incarcerated in the Philadelphia prison system, and they had been used as research material for a dizzying assortment of medical experiments. While some were embarrassed by their history as caged guinea pigs and remained silent, others were morally outraged and emotionally recounted their experiences. More than a few expressed their lasting enmity for those who had used them in such a cavalier fashion.

Over the years I would bring a number of these men and women into my classes at Temple University. Students, in most cases learning for the first time about similar episodes of unethical medical research at places such as Tuskegee, Fernald, and Willowbrook, were normally stunned by the former inmate/test subject's stories. One of the most compelling presenters was Edward Anthony. Though shy and cognizant of his modest public speaking abilities, Anthony's honest, unembellished account of his days as an imprisoned test subject held listeners' undivided attention. Facial expressions denoting shock and revulsion became commonplace; it was clear students were not listening to an ordinary guest lecturer.

Gradually, I recognized that Edward Anthony's powerful testimony of life as a test subject was worthy of a larger audience than my few Urban Society classes. For his many years of recounting his story in my own classes, our trips to other college campuses, and for his participation in this book project, I would like to offer him my sincere appreciation.

I would also like to thank Drs. Ackerman, Franzblau, and Egilman for being such fine medical role models and for ceaselessly trumpeting the importance of ethics in medicine.

The process of converting a manuscript to a prominent place on bookstore shelves is a team exercise. I am fortunate to have had the assistance of a very fine team. Sandy Thatcher, director of Penn State University Press, quickly recognized the historical importance of Eddie Anthony's story. I would like to thank the cadre of book lovers at the Press in editorial and design for their work.

I also owe a debt of gratitude to my relentless and indefatigable copyeditor. Suzanne Wolk endured my syntactical blunders, tired prose, and frenetic schedule, because she, too, recognized the importance of Ed Anthony's story.

I would also like to thank Temple's Urban Archives for their assistance with Holmesburg photographs, and Louis Edinger and George Holmes for their important contribution to this book.

x

One of the nicest [American] scientists I know was heard to say, "Criminals in our penitentiaries are fine experimental material—and much cheaper than chimpanzees."
—"Pertinax," *British Medical Journal*, January 1963

In 1998, Allen Hornblum published *Acres of Skin*, which powerfully documented the wide spectrum of abusive medical experimentation conducted at Philadelphia's Holmesburg Prison complex by Dr. Albert M. Kligman between the 1950s and 1970s. By drawing back the veil obscuring the medical abuse of captive men, Allen has done a great service not only to the abused subjects but also to all Americans by allowing them to witness the questionable milieu in which prison experimentation has been conducted.

Seventy-five percent of Holmesburg's inmate population, including Edward "Butch" Anthony, the subject of this book, were administered cosmetics, powders, and shampoos that caused many of them baldness, extensive scarring, and permanent skin and nail injury. Fingernails were removed or deformed and the subjects' backs were covered in checkerboard patterns of flayed, discolored, and scarred skin. Jailed subjects were also inoculated with herpes, vaccinia, and wart viruses. Dow Chemical Company also paid Kligman to test the suspected carcinogen dioxin, on seventy prisoners, mostly black. "Most of this research was practiced upon African American men," revealed Hornblum. "It was not uncommon for them to be used for the worst, most dangerous experiments."

Kligman, a dermatologist, was initially invited to Holmesburg Prison in 1951 to treat an outbreak of athlete's foot. But his initial reaction to Holmesburg was far from therapeutic and gave Hornblum's book its title: "All I saw before me were acres of skin. It was like a farmer seeing a fertile field for the first time." Soon Kligman was inducing foot fungus, instead of treating it, because he saw the opportunity to conduct lucrative experiments upon thousands of captive bodies for at least thirty-three major pharmaceutical and cosmetic companies, such as Johnson & Johnson, Merck, Helena Rubenstein, and DuPont.

During World War II, prisoners had been commonly used as research subjects and, after the war, the United States was the only nation in the world continuing to legally use prisoners in clinical trials. This corporate capital catalyzed a thirty-year boom in research with prisoners, and throughout the 1950s and 1960s Kligman gained exclusive experimental use of inmate bodies, testing 153 experimental drugs between 1962 and 1966 alone.

Each participant earned anywhere from ten to seven hundred dollars, while Kligman made millions for himself, the university, and his pharmaceutical partners. As Hornblum notes in *Acres of Skin,* when Kligman used prisoners to devise the anti-acne medication. Retina-A, it alone made him a millionaire. "It was years before the authorities knew that I was conducting various studies on prisoner volunteers," recalls Kligman. "Things were simple then. Informed consent was unheard of. No one asked me what I was doing. It was a wonderful time."

Far from being castigated for the harms visited on prisoners, Kligman has been honored for elevating the specialty of dermatology. But he did not confine his research to his specialty. Kligman oversaw research into many hazardous agents, including Army and CIA mind-control experiments in which men were given experimental psychoactives and Schedule II drugs (those with a high abuse risk). Some men insist that they have never recovered from these experiences.

The men of Holmesburg prison were not alone. In 1952, Chester M. Southam of the Sloan-Kettering Institute injected at least 396 inmates at Ohio State Prison—more than 180 of them black—with live human cancer cells — years before the similar and infamous Jewish Chronic Disease Hospital experiments. Between 1963 and 1971, a Dr. Heller irradiated the gonads of 131 prisoners in Oregon, including at least 66 "negro volunteers," with radioactive thymidine. Inmates also were used in flawed, unhygienic, blood-plasma trials testing "high-volume plasmapheresis"—transfusions utilizing large amounts of plasma—between 1967 and 1969 throughout the state of Alabama. Austin R. Stough, the doctor who performed these experiments, also made millions.

Informed consent is always questionable in the prison arena, where subjects have already lost their most important civil rights and where literacy is so low that the presence of a signed consent form signifies little. Allen also reminds us that prison have been closed to mainstream American society, making the *sub rosa* medical exploitation of prisoners something that could be conducted on the powerless in secret.

Recognizing this, the Ethical Committee of the World Medical Association, in its 1961 code of ethics on human experimentation, declared, "Persons detained in prisons, penitentiaries, or reformatories— being 'captive groups'—should not be used as subjects of human experiments." But in American prisons research thrived and prisoners' desperate need for money— to purchase everything from toiletries to freedom in the form of bail money—means that paying the incarcerated far more for medical research than they could earn elsewhere constitutes undue inducement or even coercion.

However, by the 1970s, research in prisons began to disappear, succumbing to scandals that unmasked the racially unbalanced, abusive, dangerous, and scientifically sloppy nature of experimentation with prisoners. The exploitation of large numbers of black male prisoners caused public-relations problems for researchers and institutions in the wake of the increasingly violent and bitter civil rights battles and the revelations of the "Tuskegee syphilis study," in which effective treatment was withheld from about four hundred poor black sharecroppers with syphilis. The deaths of twenty-nine inmates and at least ten white authority figures in the 1971 Attica prison riot sent a chill through prison medical research programs and so did the burgeoning influence of the Black Muslims who emerged as powerful critics of prison research, dissuading black inmates from participating and intimidating the overwhelmingly white medical researchers.

Research programs suffered legal repercussions, as well when, in 1979, nine Oregon prison subjects sued and shared $2,215 in damages. A January 1973 *Atlantic Monthly* story by investigative journalist Jessica Mitford uncovered the exploitative nature of prison medical research and Senator Edward Kennedy held hearings that led to the National Commission for the Protection of Biomedical and Behavioral Research (CPBBR), which investigated medical experimentation on prisoners. It considered banning such research outright, but settled instead upon sharply curtailing medical research— which all but disappeared in prisons. The 1979 Belmont Report, placed the onus on researchers for ensuring that research with prisoners provided informed consent and is therapeutic under what is called the "Common Rule": this set strict limits on nontherapeutic research and research done with prisoners and requires the review of proposed studies by institutional review boards.

When Allen published *Acres of Skin*, many former subjects realized for the first time that they had rights as experimental subjects and could sue the University of Pennsylvania, Kligman's home institution, despite the indemnification waivers that some had signed. In September 2000, 298 former Holmesburg prisoners filed a class-action lawsuit against the university, Johnson & Johnson, Dow Chemical Company, Dr. Kligman and the City of Philadelphia. But the years and the experiments had taken their physical toll. Most subjects are dead, and the survivors, now in their sixties and seventies, suffer from skin and nail problems, breathing difficulties, cancers, and stubborn, sometimes unidentified infections. Former inmates have joined as the Experimentation Survivors and Allen remains their vocal advocate.

Today, most people don't realize that prison medical research is enjoying a quiet renaissance. Since the late 1980s, prison research has been planned and conducted in Arkansas, Maryland, South Carolina, Texas, Florida, Connecticut, and Rhode Island.

In 2006 the Institute of Medicine, which advises the federal government on biomedical issues, appointed the Committee on Ethical Considerations for Protection of Prisoners Involved in Research to study the issue and recommended that prisons again be opened widely to medical research. If the doors are flung wide to investigators, will they admit therapy or exploitation? Allen's work has served an important purpose in demonstrating that the laws enacted to protect prisoners' rights and health consistently have failed to do so.

Now, in *Sentenced to Science*, Allen Hornblum expounds on this hidden history by crafting a narrative that details one man's odyssey in Holmesburg's stygian scientific kingdom. I hope it may serve as a cautionary tale.

Harriet A. Washington
Author, *Medical Apartheid*

"My Back Is on Fire"

"There were three of us in a cell at the time. I had been in the jail only a few days and had just gotten assigned to work in the tailor shop. They make socks, underwear, and other clothing for the inmates, but I hadn't actually started to work yet, so I thought I could take my time that morning while my cell buddies left for their jobs. But I soon heard my name being called out on the block. It was time for guys who had signed up for the medical tests to go down to H block.

"By then I wasn't too afraid of the experiments. My homeys said they had taken care of me and I'd be okay. They said they had made sure I wouldn't be put on any of the experiments where I'd get hurt. They told me I'd be able to make some money and wouldn't be hurt too bad. To tell the truth, I was more afraid of being sexually assaulted down there than the experiments. I had heard all sorts of bad shit about guys getting solicited for sex and fucked down on H block.

"I got my pass to get off of G block where I was celled and went over to H block, where the University of Pennsylvania doctors were doing their tests. The guard opened the gate and let us in. There must have been about twenty of us. We were all looking around, checking things out, trying not to look concerned.

"You could see where cell walls had been broken out to make larger rooms for the doctors to do their research experiments. Strange-looking medical equipment was all over the place. There were a bunch of doctors walking around doing stuff, but then I realized the guys in white smocks weren't doctors at all, but inmates. There were inmates doing all the work. In a way I felt better. I thought the tests couldn't be that bad if they had prisoners doing them. If the experiments were really something serious, I would've seen more real doctors on the block.

1

"An inmate took my pass and checked my name off on a clipboard he was holding. He directed some of us, about five or six, to a room and told me to sit on a stool and to take my shirt off. They then gave me a paper to read and told me to sign it. It basically said if anything should happen to me I'm not going to hold the University of Pennsylvania responsible.

"I said, 'Hey, why you giving me this? I thought these tests were safe.'

"'They are,' said the inmate. 'It's just a formality.'

"He said it was a bubble bath test for Johnson & Johnson and they were testing it to see if it's harmful to someone with an open wound. He said the test would run about two or three weeks and we'd make about $37. The money sounded good to me. I signed my name on the paper.

"One of these inmates in a white lab coat comes over to me and tells me to lean forward and then starts to put fresh tape on my back and then just as quickly pulls it off. He did this over and over again. He must have done it eight or ten times until he had pulled the first layer of skin off. He did this to six different spots on my back. He then got an eye dropper and put it in a little glass jar and drew up some of the solution that was in there, the bubble bath I guess, and then squeezed some of it onto a small, square gauze pad. He then placed the gauze pad on one of the spots he had just rubbed raw and taped it onto my back. He did this to each one of the six spots on my back.

"Then he placed a larger piece of tape over each spot, and I'm thinking, this ain't too bad. I can handle this. He tells me we're just about done, and I'm not feeling any pain or anything. I'm thinking my guys really took care of me. I'm making money for nothing. The inmate then picked up a green spray can and starts to spray my entire back.

"I asked what he was doing and he said, 'Oh, it ain't nothing. This is just to ensure that the patches stay on your back. It'll keep your pores closed.'

"It was sure something, though, 'cause as soon as the spray hit my back it was cold and I began to taste it in my mouth. It tasted bitter and I swear I could feel it seeping in my body. I thought it was toxic or something 'cause I started to feel dizzy.

"'Man, what the fuck is that stuff?' I said.

"He didn't say anything and started to put large pieces of tape on each side of my back. 'If this come off,' he said, 'you don't get any money.'

"I was really getting dizzy. It tasted like mentholated alcohol. My tongue was beginning to get cold like my back. It was all making me feel really nauseous.

"The inmate in the white smock doing this to me said we were done and goes on to say he'd call me down the next morning to change the bandages. He then sends me back to my cell block. While crossing center I'm feeling even more nauseous. I get onto G block and wobble to my cell with this disgusting taste in my mouth and all this stuff on my back, and as soon as I lift my leg to step in my cell I fell out. I passed right out.

"When I came to, Youngie and Ruben, my cell mates, are putting water on my face and helping me to my bunk. That's when I screamed out, 'Man, my fuckin' back is on fire. It's killing me. Fuck this test. Take this shit off my back.'

"Ruben tried to calm me down. 'Butch, you can't do that,' he said. 'If you take this shit off, you won't get paid.'

"'I don't give a shit, man,' I cried out. 'My back is on fire. It's burning the hell out of me. Get it the fuck off. It's killing me.'

"'Don't worry,' says Youngie, 'I'll hook you up.'

"He then carefully peeled off the tape sealer and taped the upper edges of it to the cell wall. Then he took the smaller patches off and stuck them on the wall as well. He said that's what everyone does who is having a bad reaction but still wants to earn that money. I didn't give a shit about the money at that point, though, 'cause my back was screaming. I really felt like my back was on fire.

"Youngie then got a bucket of water from the shower room and washed my back with soap and water. There was little relief, though. My back burned all night long. I'm thinking hour after hour, 'What the hell did I do to myself? What did those damn people do to me?'

"When morning finally comes, I can't wait to see a doctor and have this thing taken care of, but Youngie tells me he's got to hook me up first. He says he got to put that shit back on me, so I'll be ready when they call me. He was thinkin' more about the money than I was. I just wanted the pain to end. I tell you, I'm countin' the seconds.

"I get out of bed and turn around for the patches to be put back on, and Youngie says to Ruben, 'Damn, look at this shit here.'

"'Man,' says Ruben, 'that's some nasty-lookin' shit. Whadda they do to you?'

"I couldn't see what they were talkin' about, but I sure as hell could feel it.

"Large blisters the size of nickels and filled with pus had formed where the patches had been. I just shook my head at the mess I had gotten myself into. I was weak, in pain, and my back had this constant burning.

"My Back Is on Fire"

"The block runner came down with my pass and I went over to H block. I was hoping to see a doctor, but it was the same ol' inmate in a white lab jacket who looked at me. All he said was, 'Wow,' when he saw my back.

"'Does this normally happen?' I asked him.

"'Sometimes,' was all he replied. He grabbed what looked like a pair of tweezers and a little scalpel-type instrument and cut the blisters off and drained the pus outta the wounds. He then cleaned each of the six blistered areas, put new patches on, and sprayed the area once again before putting large swathes of tape on. That same chemical taste filled my mouth, but I didn't get as nauseous this time, just a little lightheaded. As I'm walking back to my block I'm wondering when this pain is gonna subside. The blisters were cut off, but my back still felt like it was on fire.

"I got back to my cell and the guys helped me take the shit off again. They washed my back, but it still felt like I was lying on hot coals. There was no relief; it was terrible. All day and all night I'm in pain. I ain't getting no sleep. I'm moaning and keeping the other guys from getting any sleep. I'm really feelin' miserable, and now a new problem comes up. My back is turning red, as red as a strawberry. The blisters didn't come back, but now I'm a black guy with a fire-engine-red back. And it still feels like it's on fire.

"On the third day I get a pass to go down to H block, and once again I see this inmate doctor or whatever he's supposed to be and say to him, 'Don't you have the results of this goddamn test yet? My back is on fire. Look man, I can't take any more of this shit. You guys are killing me. Look at my back. It's blood red. I want you to take care of this shit now.'

"The inmate knew I was serious this time and was probably afraid I was gonna hurt 'im, so he went down the block and talked to a University of Pennsylvania doctor, a short, light-skinned black guy in a suit and tie. He comes over to me and I show him my back.

"'Hmm,' he says, lookin' all puzzled and shit. 'Look,' he says, 'I tell you what. You can take the patches off. You don't have to wear them anymore.'

"'You throwing me off the test?' I ask him.

"'Under the circumstances it may be for the best.'

"'What about my money,' I said, concerned they might try to cheat me.

"'You'll get paid. We'll make sure you get the full amount that's coming to you.'

"As I'm walking back to my block I'm feeling somewhat relieved that I'm off the test and still gonna get paid, but then I realize my back is still killing me. The doctor didn't treat me at all. He didn't do shit. The motherfucker didn't even give me anything for the pain. They were just a bunch of sadists.

"All that day and into the night it starts getting worse. It was unbearable. My whole fuckin' body is reacting. It was like something was crawling under my skin. Under my arms and between my legs it's getting real hot. I'm moaning. My cell mates can't do anything for me, and I'm keeping them from getting any sleep at night. I'm thinking the whole time, what the hell did I get myself into? I'm blaming my cell partners, the damn doctors, myself, I don't know who to blame.

"The only thing that seemed to relieve the itching and the pain was hot showers. I mean, real hot. Guys couldn't believe I was able to stand under scalding hot water like I was, but it was the only thing that eased the pain and itching. They must have thought I was losing my mind. The nights were terrible, though; I just laid there in agony.

"The next morning Ruben and Youngie look at me and can't believe their eyes. I got fine little red bumps all over my face, arms, legs, head, chest, all over. Some were white and filled with pus. The guys thought I had German measles or some dreaded tropical disease.

"Youngie tells the block guard I'm messed up bad and got to see one of the H block doctors, but the turnkey comes back and tells us I'm off the tests. He can't send me down to the Penn research unit. I can't believe what's happening to me. I'm in pain. I look like a goddamn strawberry. And now I'm off the tests and the doctors won't even look at me. Youngie and me start raising a ruckus, demanding I see a doctor, and the guard says he'll see what he can do. In the meantime, he tells me to go down to the visiting room. He says I got a visit.

"That's when I really found out just how bad I looked. You don't have any mirrors in prison, so I didn't really know what I looked like. That visit told me just how bad things had gotten.

"My sister Edna had come up to Holmesburg to see me. She was already seated behind the screen when I got to the visiting booth. She took one look at me and started screaming. She jumped out of her chair in horror. She was jumping up and down, yelling, 'Oh my God, oh my God, what did they do to you?' She was holding her hand to her mouth like she was trying to keep from vomiting.

"The guards immediately rushed me and tackled me to the floor. They thought I had done something to her to cause such a commotion. Edna started to yell at them, 'Stop, he didn't do anything. Leave him alone. He didn't do anything. Can't you see he's hurt? Look at him. Leave him alone.'

"They let me get up. Edna was still hysterical and started yelling, 'What the hell did they do to you? What are they doing to you in here?'

"I told her, 'I got on the tests.'

"'What tests?' she asked. 'What are you talking about? What kinds of tests do something like that? Is you crazy?'

"I told her I needed the money. Nobody at home was sending me anything.

"She said, 'Don't get on any more tests. We'll send you money. Promise you won't get on any more of those tests. They're killing you.'

"It was pretty bad. The thing with my sister really shook me up. Back on the block, me and Youngie are still tryin' to get the guard to give me a pass to go down to H block to get checked out. The guard can see for himself I'm in need of medical attention. He tells me to go down to the chow hall for breakfast and he'll try to have some news for me by the time I get back.

"But when I get down to the chow hall everybody starts staring at me and making comments and moving away. They're looking at these little bumps on my face and arms and how red I am. Guys don't want to get too close to me. They don't want me next to them in the chow line. They think I got some deadly disease and they're goin' to catch it. They tell me to get the hell away from them. Some of 'em start threatening me if I get too close. Even the cooks and kitchen workers start eyeballing me and aren't sure if they should serve me. They're thinking just by putting that mush on my plate they're serving they're gonna get contaminated.

"Finally a guard comes over to me and says, 'What the fuck is wrong with you?'

"I tell him, 'I got on the tests.'

"He called me a stupid motherfucker, and said, 'Look man, you better take it on the hop. Better take your sick ass outta here before you cause something to jump off.'

"'But whaddabout my food?'

"He says, 'I'll have a cook make up a platter for you and send it to your block.'

"Man, can you believe it? I couldn't even go down to the mess hall now. They didn't want a disturbance with me lookin' the way I did and said they'd send my food to my cell. It was that bad.

"Back in my cell I'm still in pain. It feels like something is crawling under my skin. The itching was terrible. My armpits and groin are startin' to heat up and be on fire like my back. I couldn't keep my arms down by my side and I'm having trouble walking. Any sort of movement hurts. And I'm wondering if it can get any worse.

"I was an introvert. I never wanted to stand out or draw attention to myself and now I look like a neon sign. I can't believe what those Penn doctors did to me. I'm thinkin' those doctors gave me some toxic poison and now I'm all fucked up. Maybe dying. What the hell did they do to me?"

Twenty years old and already a veteran of illicit drugs, gang wars, and the ever-present and explosive street violence that is so common to life in the "hood," Edward "Butch" Anthony was reaping a health crisis of unimaginable proportions—all due to his decision to become a human guinea pig. What had been described as a "safe and easy" way to earn a few dollars while incarcerated in a big-city jail had become a physical and psychological nightmare. Literally overnight, Butch Anthony, a healthy, vibrant black man and survivor of one of the most unforgiving ghettos in America, had unknowingly embarked on a confidence-searing and health-shattering journey as harrowing as any landmine-laden trip one could envision.

As a test subject in Holmesburg Prison's medical research program in the mid-1960s, he would become a particularly unlucky experimental lab rat.[1] Probed with needles transferring mysterious solutions, bathed in strange chemicals, and paid to swallow experimental compounds, Anthony—by his own admission a "functional illiterate"—was a most receptive and compliant guinea pig for hire. An unquestioning dollar-a-day human vessel willing to endure a barrage of physical affronts, not to mention a paternalistic relationship with single-minded researchers that only former prisoner test subjects could truly understand. The upshot was a series of strange and inexplicable medical maladies and conundrums that would last a lifetime.

Although the physical problems Anthony accumulated in these experiments were considerable, and his repeated decisions to become "a brother for science" difficult to comprehend, one can be assured he was not alone—there were thousands of desperate, incarcerated men and women just like him in postwar America. Imprisoned Americans who shockingly discovered that they had not only been sentenced to prison, but sentenced to science as well.

And for the vast majority of these formerly imprisoned test subjects—in addition to the scars and regrets—there remains a lasting enmity toward doctors, hospitals, and the medical establishment in general. This residual skepticism—antipathy would be more accurate—toward physicians and medical researchers is especially prominent in the African American community.[2] Past revelations surrounding the infamous Tuskegee syphilis study, combined with their own personal indignities and the more recent revelations regarding the Holmesburg Prison medical experiments, have left several generations of black Americans with a profound distrust of the American medical establishment. For the many black Philadelphians who had loved ones in Holmesburg, the cynicism is practically palpable.

Butch Anthony's story is more than a tale of physical torment and personal failure—an urban melodrama focusing on one individual's descent into drugs, crime, and imprisonment. More important, it is also a cautionary tale for a proud, prosperous nation that espouses democratic principles and egalitarian notions of fairness and justice but for far too long found it convenient to use its weakest, most vulnerable populations—the retarded, the indigent, orphans, and prisoners—as raw material for medical experimentation.[3]

Anthony, no doubt, has to shoulder the burden for his own self-destructive decisions and troubled behavior. But America has some self-assessment to do as well. The nation has yet to truly grapple with its own sordid history of using people as throwaway objects, and with the wide chasm between lofty proclamations of honorable goals and ethical conduct and the many embarrassing acts of greed, self-interest, and cavalier behavior that have pockmarked our history.

Butch Anthony's story reveals the dark underbelly of American medicine. And though his personal account may prove an uncomfortable revelation to many unaware of the treatment accorded warehoused individuals during the second half of the twentieth century, he was not alone—there were many others like him. Nameless, faceless institutionalized test subjects, human grist for the research mill that a God-fearing, freedom-loving, but uninterested country repeatedly turned its back on. Anthony's story is their story, and it is long overdue that we allow at least one of them to voice what it was like to be an incarcerated human guinea pig.

"The Jungle"

It may have been a momentary slip of the tongue or just an offhand remark at a particularly trying time, but its racial bite and cultural impact on the urban lexicon of the third-largest city in America would last a generation or more. There can be little doubt that Police Commissioner Thomas J. Gibbons's reference, in the mid-1950s, to a large swath of North Philadelphia as "the jungle" wasn't necessarily intended to stigmatize a struggling section of the city as a ruthless, cutthroat piece of real estate inhabited by a lesser species, but eventually the racially charged sobriquet caught on.[1]

The negative handle stuck like paper on glue, and for decades thereafter the pejorative term for North Philadelphia seemed impossible to shed.

In all likelihood, in fact, it was probably a freelance article by a former newspaper writer and local television director that did more to popularize the term than the frank comments of a beleaguered police commissioner. The 1957 *Sunday Bulletin* article, entitled "The Jungle: Seven Square Miles That Shame—and Menace—Our City," set off a firestorm of indignation and moral outrage from those who resided within the boundaries of "Poplar Street north to Lehigh Avenue and from the Delaware River west to the Schuylkill."

Described as "dark and dense and dreary" as well as "dismal and dangerous," the "jungle," according to the author of the provocative essay, was "Philadelphia's shame and sorrow. Philadelphia's greatest menace and Philadelphia's greatest challenge." Highlighting such issues as neighborhood "squalor" and "density," "dilapidated houses," and "crimes per month," the author argued that "the problems posed by the jungle cause our wisest men to shake their heads, lower their eyes and sigh, then look you straight in the eye and say with grim determination, 'If we can't solve this problem, we don't deserve to have a city.'"[2]

2

Though there was much that was good in the area—numerous "neat and tidy streets with freshly scrubbed marble doorsteps" owned by pleasant, considerate neighbors—there was overwhelming evidence that much was wrong, troubling, and inhospitable about the place. Regrettably, within just a few minutes of Philadelphia's grand and majestic City Hall lay a totally different world.

According to the article, this primitive and unforgiving piece of terrain could be reached easily; one need only travel north on Broad Street, "and at any point in the seventeen blocks between Poplar Street and Lehigh Avenue turning to the right or left" one could find "overcrowded tenements, garish taprooms, squalid speakeasies, debris-littered streets," and a wide array of criminal behavior.[3]

It hadn't always been that way. The neighborhoods throughout this portion of the city were once a rich mix of handsome estates, middle-class row homes, and smaller versions of the same that surrounded factories manufacturing everything from ships and locomotives to textiles and electronics. Communities from one river to the other thrived. "Where one family once lived in elegance," however, "four to six families now live in squalor. One bed is enough for as many as four children. One bedroom is enough for an entire family—mother, father and children. But despite this lack of privacy, children are conceived and born with great frequency."

Not surprisingly, "the forest of dilapidated houses," trash-strewn streets, and overpopulation contributed to a soaring crime rate. The North Central Police District, for example, had an average of 612 major crimes a month, more than a hundred above its closest rival and several hundred more than the better sections of the city. Violent crime had become a way of life—and death—in the area.

The "jungle" article provoked considerable controversy and precipitated a long-running public debate over both the article's accuracy and various remediation proposals to fix this growing blight on the city's image.[4] Some commentators quibbled over the jungle's boundaries, only to conclude, "I wouldn't go through that area if my life depended on it."[5] Others denounced the article as perpetuating a "myth that the African culture, devastated by four hundred years of slave trade, was a late Stone Age culture no better than that of the American Indian."[6] A few laid "the cancerous growth" at the feet of a series of incompetent city administrations, while others sought out root causes, arguing that "ignorance, folly, alcohol, poverty, immorality, illegitimacy," among other factors, were "breeding the criminals of tomorrow in these cesspools of shame."[7]

Despite all the editorial verbiage, dueling op-ed pieces, town meetings, and community initiatives, the jungle's many-faceted problems continued to grow. One of the more visible and threatening developments was the stunning increase in gang violence. It was as if corner hangouts consisting of aimless, hopeless teenagers had become independent medieval fiefdoms or warlike nations during a time of universal strife, each protecting its turf as if the lives of its members depended upon it—and they usually did. For the next decade and a half, scores of teenage boys would have their lives terminated by gang wars. One mayoral administration counted forty-five "juvenile gangs" in the jungle comprising more than two thousand members, and further categorized eight of the gangs "as the most vicious in the city," accounting for more than 3,100 arrests in just one year.[8]

As violent confrontations between the DeMarcos, the Vikings, Camac & Diamond, the Valley, the Tenderloin, and the dozens of other gangs in the area escalated over the years, the salient facts and death toll from these bloody skirmishes were recorded as if they were the highlights of a Phillies ballgame. As one *Evening Bulletin* article headline read— almost as if in numerical code—"2–4 Shoots 2–8 at Corner of 2–7."[9] The article went on to explain that an eighteen-year-old boy standing on the corner of 27th and Master with three friends was approached by six youths, one of whom yelled out, "Two-four here," and pulled out a sawed-off shotgun from under his coat and shot the youth. Though only a few blocks apart, the "24th Street Gang" and the "28th Street Gang" were deadly enemies.

Gang life was certifiably dangerous, as the city medical examiner could attest, but it didn't slow the recruitment process. As one North Philly gang member admitted, "I wanted to be from a gang. I guess it's because gang members are known to be hard, all of them can fight, they stay out all night, they drink wine and many other things. But the main reason is because it felt good to belong to someone. The only real thing a person has to relate to is the gangs."[10]

That sense of community, however tribal and warlike in its orientation, came at a steep price. For a young man in his teens, growing up in the jungle was a daily challenge. Just walking down the street could turn into a life-threatening adventure. Edward Anthony was one of those boys.

11

The word itself can easily conjure pastoral visions of rolling hills, meandering streams, and lush valleys. Landscaped countryside encompassing quaint little towns, white church steeples, country inns. But the "Village" of Eddie Anthony's youth is a far cry from that serene, bucolic image. In fact, Anthony's village is a crowded, trash-strewn urban battleground that produced more tears, bloodshed, and regrets than fond remembrances. For a sensitive and shy youth balancing demanding, Bible-toting parents and high-spirited, combative community elements, the Village was serious culture shock—life on the street appeared to be more a primer for societal mayhem than a cherished guidebook for simple and sober living.

Bounded by Lehigh Avenue on the north, 22nd Street on the east, 34th Street on the west, and Diamond Street on the south, the Village sat prominently in almost the geographical center of North Philadelphia. The community had once been exclusively white and of mixed European ethnicity. By the time of Edward Anthony's birth on August 19, 1943, at Hahnemann Hospital, the neighborhood surrounding his home at 2321 North 27th Street was taking on a decidedly darker cast. Thousands of black families from the Deep South had been moving to northern industrial cities like Detroit, Chicago, Gary, New York, and Newark in search of a better life, and the Anthony family of Augusta, Georgia, was among them.

Edward's parents, Joseph Anthony, a cement finisher and laborer, and his mother, Julia Schley, a housewife and devout church member, came to Pennsylvania in the early 1930s during the first great black migration. They settled in Philadelphia, on 27th Street between York and Dauphin streets, and would eventually raise nine children, little Edward—or Butch, as he would come to be known—being the last and most coddled of the brood. His older brothers—Joe, Tommy, and Wilbert—and his sisters— Lucille, Karribelle, Edna, Marlene, and Alease—would dote on their youngest sibling and, along with their parents' overprotective nature, would play a significant role in shaping Edward's confused outlook on his immediate surroundings and the world beyond.

In addition to Edward's large family, the neighborhood he grew up in would have a critical role in shaping his life. A racially mixed community during Anthony's formative years in the early 1950s, Strawberry Mansion, or the white section of the Village that bordered Fairmount Park and ran from 29th to 34th Street, would become almost entirely African American by the end of the decade. Demographic shifts in Philly's residential makeup would cause sweeping changes in many urban neighborhoods, including the Mansion, once the province of a vibrant, largely Jewish middle class, which saw a mass exodus of Jewish families during these years.

Though he was probably too young to fully appreciate the significant racial and economic changes taking place in his own backyard, Butch Anthony was already struggling with a host of issues. Race, however, was not one of them.

"There were white boys sitting in my house all the time when I was a kid growing up, but I was never allowed to go to their homes. My mother was scared of white people. She was brought up in the South. She'd tell me, 'When school is over you come right home. And don't go to anybody's house.' She said it was okay if the white boys from McIntyre Elementary School at 30th and Gordon wanted to come to my house, but I wasn't ever allowed to go to theirs.

"My parents were very strict with me. I wasn't allowed to do a lot of stuff that other kids were doing. It seemed that my brothers could be free and frolic as they wished, but I was always being protected and punished for a lot of things that others were allowed to do. That whole situation was terrible and used to drive me crazy.

"We had a very close and respected family in the community. My father was a strict Baptist deacon of the church and my mom was the secretary and treasurer of the church. The church was a very big part of my family's life. Me and my sisters had to attend choir practice and Bible school several days during the week and go to church every Sunday. The church was at 28th and Dauphin and the Reverend Davis Debrady was our pastor. He lived five houses down the street from us, and that made it all the worse. His sermons scared me. I hated being threatened with fire and brimstone at every sermon. It really gave me a messed-up conception of God and what a righteous life was supposed to be like. You weren't supposed to do this and you weren't supposed to do that. And if you did any of these things, bad stuff would happen to you. It was really messed up. I was scared all the time, and my brothers and sisters tried to keep me scared. It was a game to them. I was too shy and sensitive. And judging from the rough neighborhood I was growing up in, my parents' philosophy and religious beliefs didn't make any sense.

"In my house I was brought up with discipline and usually overprotected. But around the corner and on the lots we played at, all hell was

13

breaking loose. There were always lots of fights. Fights on the way to school. Fights on the way back from school. Going to the movies, going to the store. You had to be ready to fight 'cause you knew you were gonna be threatened. My sister Alease, who was five years older than me, had to walk me to school every day 'cause my parents thought I'd get picked on and end up in a fight. They were always trying to protect me from negative things in the neighborhood, but their pampering me drove me crazy. It only made things worse.

"I remember sitting on the front step one time when I was a little kid, and I got into a whole lot of trouble for just defending myself. My mother wouldn't let me go off and play with the other kids. She thought she was keeping me safe by keeping me from the neighborhood. She'd tell me to just sit on the front steps and not get pulled into anything she or I would be ashamed of. Well, don't you know, a couple kids come by and start calling me a sissy because I won't leave the front of the house. I wouldn't leave the steps. One of 'em, Charles Tucker, soon calls me a sissy-assed motherfucker and starts a fight with me. We're taking shots at each other and I'm trying to defend my honor, and my mother comes out, breaks up the fight, and punishes me for getting off the steps and fighting. She whipped my ass pretty good, but I was only tryin' to defend myself. I was so angry I wanted to kill her.

"It was stuff like that that drove me nuts. My brothers are teaching me how to box and showing me how to get stronger by doing push-ups and sit-ups and not take any shit from anybody, but my parents are raising me to be a goody two-shoes in one of the fightinest neighborhoods in the city. Trying to live with these different attitudes and philosophies was a constant struggle. I didn't know which way to go. Just trying to figure what was right and what was wrong wore me out.

"Everybody in the Village knew my family. My parents and brothers and sisters were well liked. Everybody seemed to know each other. Right around the corner from us was 2800 York Street, and everyone who lived there was from Georgia. They all knew each other from down South. We called those blocks of York and Susquehanna Avenue Little Georgia 'cause everybody came from there. It was all like family. Parents back then seemed to watch over kids more than they do today, even if the kids weren't theirs. Sometimes it was like you had three or four sets of parents watching over you.

"My father worked two and three jobs and we never lacked anything. We always had enough in the way of food and clothing. We were one of the first families on the street to have a television in the fifties, and people used to line up on the sidewalk and peek through the windows to get a look at popular comedy shows like *Amos and Andy*. Years later, when color televisions came out, we figured out a way to have our own homemade color TV. We used to put a piece of blue, yellow, or orange plastic over the TV screen to make it look like we had a color TV in our house.

"My parents were religious and very strict, especially with me. They didn't believe in sparing the rod. My father had a leather cat-o'-nine tails and he'd whip us good when we were bad. Parents in the neighborhood liked and trusted me. They let their kids come out and play with me when they wouldn't with some other kids in the neighborhood. They knew my parents had raised me right. When we were kids, we couldn't wait to get out of our parents' eyesight so we could curse and act like the older jitter-bugs in our neighborhood.

"As time went on, life in the Village got a lot rougher. There were a lot of gangs, and fights and fair ones were occurring all the time. All of my older brothers could fight, but my oldest brother, Joe, who was twenty-five years older than me, was a killer. He had been a professional fighter and belonged to the Village Dukes Boxing Club that had guys like Georgie Benton, Gill Turner, and Beau Jack working out and training there. All of my brothers were over six feet tall and could box, but Joe was the best. He was a heavyweight and fought over two hundred exhibitions against Joe Louis when they were in the service together. They would just go around to different army bases and put on boxing exhibitions to entertain the troops. My brother Joe was somebody you really didn't want to mess with.

"But Joe wasn't the only tough guy in the neighborhood. There were a lot of 'em, and those niggers could fight. Guys like Junie Harley, Clayton Schley, and the Blunt brothers were some serious niggers. Junie Harley could fight his ass off, and the Blunt brothers were some of the baddest niggers in the Village. You had to learn how to fight and have some boys with you, or else you were gonna be in a world of hurt. That neighborhood was deep. You had to be in a gang."

As a child growing up in the heart of the jungle, Eddie Anthony was understandably ignorant of the shifting demographics and changing socioeconomic fortunes affecting his community. The flight of white residents to Northeast Philadelphia and the suburbs and the gradual demise of the area's industrial base were beyond his comprehension.

"The Jungle"

The once noisy and frantic activity generated by the large factories and clothing manufacturers had ceased, the urban landscape was less well maintained, and the streets and empty lots he played on were more littered with trash and graffiti.

As a child, however, Butch had other things on his mind. He and his friends were busy playing handball behind the electric company on Gordon Street, buying penny candy at Jeff's Grocery Store at 27th and Dauphin, spending the afternoon at the Park Movie Theater at 31st and Diamond, speculating on the uses of interesting objects and gadgets at Brodie's Hardware Store at 25th and York, and watching the community's elders patronize the many local taprooms in the area, like the Rock and Roll Bar at 26th and York streets.

Though Butch may have been uninformed about the closure of major North Philadelphia clothing manufacturers and the economic fallout for families throughout the area, he was aware of what was happening to well-patronized neighborhood establishments within a few blocks of his home, like the Big Store, John's Bargain Store, and Libby's Clothing Store. One after the other, they started to close their doors for good. "The cleaners folded and the state store closed, and then Libby's," recalls Butch. "There was more boosting going on there like a muthafucker. Things were just walking the fuck out of those stores. They finally closed down."

Things were definitely changing. Butch was moving from single to double digits in age, and with that advance came a host of new friends, interests, and activities, many of which ran counter to his parents' expressed wishes and intentions. The fun and excitement of the streets were too much to resist, particularly for a youngster who resented the restrictive shackles of stern, religious parents. Being forced to stay home and play jacks and jump rope with his older sisters, instructed to reject what appeared fun and universally available to everyone else, and force-fed a long litany of sobering biblical teachings led to rebellion. Little Butch was growing up, and in the Village that could only mean one thing—trouble.

"Right across the street from my house was Big Red's, a horse stable that kept horses and wagons that were used by the local milkmen, icemen, and junk men that worked the area. When we thought no one was looking, me and the other kids would sneak into the stables and take off with anything we could find, leather goods, whips, clothing, whatever. Most of the time we walked off with quarts of chocolate milk, orange juice, and whole watermelons. Booze as well. The junk man used to keep a bottle of wine on his wagon for his own use, and we'd find it and get drunk. We thought we were like a lot of adults in the Village, drinking and partying. We were only seven or eight years old and would do that sort of stuff until my parents or someone else's parents would catch us. Most of us had already stolen our parents' cigarettes and experimented. We were kids on the street acting out the way kids do, especially me. I was very high strung and resented the heavy-handed approach my mother and father used to raise me. I wanted to be free to do things like everybody else. In the ghetto, people learn shit quick. Children on the street act out and are molded by watching all this shit.

"Even though they were more free to do things than me, my brothers and sisters would also feel confined by my parents' attitudes and do stuff when my mother and father left the house. When my parents used to go away for a church trip or something, my sisters used to have parties. They'd have their friends bring over beer and wine and we'd have a hell of a party. The TV would be shut off and they'd turn on the radio and listen to stations we weren't normally allowed to listen to. They'd turn up the volume and be dancing to some good jazz or rock 'n' roll that was popular at the time. They'd all be drinking and laughing and dancing, and somebody would spot me and say, 'Look at little Butch. He's dressed so cute.'

"They'd offer me a sip of wine, and then a few more sips, and would get a kick out of watching me dance and how the alcohol affected me. I'd be doing the camel walk and other dances popular at the time, and everyone would be clapping and laughing. It was fun. And I liked the feeling from drinking the wine. The dizziness relaxed me. I gradually got to like it and it helped me escape reality. I really needed something to calm me down. Most of the time I was feeling like, stop the world—I want to get off. The alcohol and then the drugs that came later allowed me to do that.

"I identified with the jitterbugs in the neighborhood. I wanted to get away from all the restraints my parents put on me and started hanging with guys who were cool and doing cool things. But I let the niggers talk me into doing things I shouldn't have been doing. I was always very susceptible to what others wanted me to do. They were stealing and fighting and drinking. I was too sensitive and usually scared of my shadow, but I went along with what they were doing. That's where the drinking helped. It took me out of all the things I was always worried about. It got me to relax. I was aware of all these dangerous situations at an early age. The violence in the Village was sometimes alley to alley, house to house, and bar to bar. There were neighborhood brawls, family feuds, and gang wars. People were getting killed when they were caught in neighborhoods where they didn't belong. North Philly was rough. You were always in danger. That's why the drinking helped. We'd save our money, and instead of buying pretzels, potato chips, and sodas, as kids do, we were getting older guys we knew to buy us quarts of wine. And we were only kids.

"We'd even be drinking in school. I went to FitzSimon's Junior High School at 26th and Huntingdon streets and we found a way to sneak half-gallon jugs of wine into the school's boiler room. We discovered a passageway in the basement that led to an unlocked door. We'd bring the jug of wine in, hide it where the maintenance people couldn't find it, and then sneak down during school and get drunk. Sometimes I'd go to my homeroom first thing in the morning, get checked in, and then play hooky the rest of the day. We'd be down in the boiler room drinking and end up going home drunk.

"We were probably drinking at school every other day. Sometimes I'd just play hooky and drink and hang out with my friends. We thought we were pretty cool. We were smoking, drinking, boxing, and wearing hats on the side of our heads like all the cool dudes in the Village. We even learned how to stroll. It was very important to have the right walk. You had to have a tough-guy stroll. My heart wasn't really into it, but if you wanted to be seen by others in the right way, you had to stroll. You had to hook your left arm and swing your right arm just so. Only sissies didn't box and stroll."

Butch Anthony was barely a teenager, but despite being protected by his devout Baptist parents and guided for better or worse by his numerous siblings, he was on a course that was destined for trouble. Lessons in Leviticus, Deuteronomy, and the wisdom of the Apostles had been replaced by cheap wine, cutting school, and joining a gang. And there would be more to learn. Now he was coming of age where the laws of the streets—particularly in the jungle—were taken more seriously. Just crossing into another group's territory could result in the most severe consequences. Physical confrontations between rival gangs of youths were bloody and occasionally deadly affairs. Gangs in the jungle—the Valley, the Demarcos, the Vikings, the Tenderloin, and the many others that had staked out a piece of dismal urban turf—were willing to bring all to bear in an effort to destroy their enemies. Guns and knives were a critical part of the arsenal.

"It was 1954 and we were into making zip guns and tack guns. We were taught by an old man, an army veteran. He even gave us gunpowder so we could protect our turf from other neighborhood gangs. All we really needed was wood, a car antenna, and a door latch, stuff that could be gotten in our daily travels. We would obtain the wood in wood shop at FitzSimons Junior High School, steal the antennas off of parked cars, and grab simple door latches whenever we spotted one in someone's house.

"At school we'd cut a block of wood in the shape of a handgun and carve a narrow path along the top where the barrel would be placed. The bottom section of an antenna worked perfectly as a barrel of a gun. Twenty-two caliber bullets passed through it perfectly. The screw would then be put in place as the trigger mechanism. Thick rubber bands were used as the trigger.

"Tack guns were similar, except we'd use one of the smaller parts of the antenna for the barrel. It would be just large enough to accommodate a tack or nail. We'd then break off match heads and crush them into powder and pack the front and back ends of the barrel. A tack or nail would be placed at the front end of the gun and we'd hold a match to the back end until it ignited. There would be a loud bang and the nail would be propelled out of the barrel at a pretty good rate of speed. There was definitely some force behind it. It could cause a great deal of pain, break the skin or cause the loss of an eye if it caught you there.

"Some guys got elaborate and made double-barreled zip guns, and I seen some that were able to fire a .38-caliber bullet. All you needed was a larger pipe to hold a larger projectile.

"I never got hurt in a gang war, but I know a number of guys who really got fucked up. There were some bitter feelings, and some guys got killed in these neighborhood fights. I saw a guy named Toothpick jump Rudy Davis one time and stab him in the head and back several times. It looked like a Watusi slaughtering an elephant. Man, it was a bloody mess. There was once a battle right outside my house where the Tenderloin came and stabbed one of our guys with a bayonet and broke the jaw of another guy. Later that night our guys got together, and you could see some of 'em were carrying Venetian blind boxes. The boxes were filled with brand-new shotguns. We got them back good.

19

"There was another time one of our guys placed a military machine gun in the trunk of his black sedan. Somebody fired a shotgun at him and he opened up with the machine gun. It was like World War II right out there in the street. Everybody was running for cover.

"The old heads were teaching the younger guys like me how to fight. Some of my own people considered me a mama's boy 'cause of the way my parents raised me, but others knew I had been taught how to fight by my older brothers. My brothers had a serious reputation in the Village, so that gave me a lot of weight in the community. But I wasn't really like them. I didn't like to rumble. I was shy and quiet, but people expected me to be out there, to take part in things and be a leader. It wasn't me, though, and the tension from trying to fill people's expectations of me always made me feel uncomfortable. My parents had pushed me in one direction and the neighborhood was pushing me in another. I felt my life was always in turmoil and I was constantly looking for a way out, searching for an answer to these deep, conflicted feelings I had.

"I finally found the answer, but it came in the form of alcohol and drugs."

"Bubble-Eyed Butch"

"We were only thirteen and fourteen years old and going to FitzSimons Junior High, but we would get ahold of a quart of wine or fifth of whiskey and get as drunk as Indians. We were drinking right in the school. And we did it every day. We'd do some gang warring, but the drinking became an everyday thing. Pretty soon I was into reefer and cough syrup, wearing a tam, and talking some hip shit—I became a damn beatnik. I converted from rock 'n' roll to jazz and dropped that damn gang stuff. We'd be talking bullshit, reading and spouting off poetry while the other crazy motherfuckers were shooting each other like dogs out in the streets.

"Drugs gave me confidence. I went from a scary-assed nigger who was as frightened as the folks you saw on *Amos and Andy* to having the devil brought out in me. I could really talk that shit and act confident when I was high on that stuff. Once I got a taste of drugs I really turned around. At 25th and Diamond and on almost any other corner in my neighborhood I could pick up some of the best reefer in the city.

"My cousin Darrell, who everyone called 'Frog,' gave me my first taste of marijuana when I was fourteen. He was only a year or two older than me, but he had already become experienced with drugs. He then just passed what he knew on to me. Initially I'd just be smoking reefer on weekends, but as time went by I wanted it every day. I really loved it. I didn't realize it at the time, but I was becoming addicted. What I did know was that I laughed more and was happier. I found the humor in things, when I was too nervous and ill at ease before. It gave me confidence to deal with people and situations that I used to have difficulty with.

"Smoking reefer even increased my appetite and improved my athletic ability. For example, I used to work out with the other guys at Champs Gym, which was at the intersection of 33rd, Dauphin, and Ridge

3

avenues. It was a real hotbed of down-and-dirty fighters. Champs was a serious blood pit. Some real tough dudes used to train there, and I was just one of the young bucks who'd be watching the veterans spar with each other and then try and imitate them when it was my turn. But when I was on reefer I could hit the bag like Joe Louis and would outrun the older guys when we were doing roadwork in Fairmount Park. Smoking reefer definitely helped me physically.

"Reefer back then cost $1 a stick or $5 for a bag that you could turn into five to ten marijuana cigarettes, depending on how you rolled them. I was smoking it every day and began selling it, but I wasn't making any money. I was still a kid, and the money didn't mean that much to me. I used to smoke my profits away. I even started to burn people by selling them reefer mixed with oregano when I smoked more of my supply than I should have. It was dangerous to shortchange customers, but fortunately nothing really bad came of it.

"One of my sisters, as it turns out, played a big role in getting me into the drug trade. She had a girlfriend in the neighborhood that had a friend in New York who was a serious marijuana dealer, and he used to send her a brick or two of the stuff to sell. She and my sister couldn't get rid of it all, so they employed me to help them move it on the street. I was selling $10 bags all over the neighborhood. Funny thing, though, I never seemed to have any money. That was okay 'cause I was always getting high."

"A year or so later, when I was around fourteen or fifteen years old, my cousin once again comes around telling me he's got something for me. He says I'm gonna love it.

"'Man, do I have something for you,' says Frog. 'I'm gonna hook you up with something that'll give you Technicolor dreams.'

"'Listen nigger,' I tell him, 'I ain't falling for that shit. You got to prove it.'

"'On Friday,' says Frog, 'if I got the money, I'm gonna hook you up. Butch, you'll be flyin' like a wild motherfucker.'

"It was an intriguing thing. I didn't really know what he was talking about, and he could have been blowing smoke up my ass, but Frog was down with enough shit that it could have been true. He definitely caught my interest.

"On Friday he came around and took me to Doc K's drugstore at Ridge and Dauphin streets. There were five Jewish pharmacies in the area, and all of 'em would sell you bennies and cough syrup if you had a connection, but Doc K's was our favorite. He goes up to Doc K, this old Jewish pharmacist who's had his shop there since the neighborhood was nothing but Jews, and asks for six ounces of Tussar. The old guy behind the counter gives us one of those skeptical looks, but pours the cough syrup and takes our money. We then went over to my aunt's house at 29th and Nicholas Street. Frog cut the Tussar in half and we each swallowed three ounces of this thick, dark liquid that looked like motor oil. It tasted awful. Almost immediately I get nauseous and feel like I'm gonna throw up. It wasn't long before I did, I began to vomit.

"'What did you do to me, man?' I yelled at Frog. 'I feel like shit. Why'd you make me drink that shit? That stuff is terrible.'

"'Relax man,' said Frog. 'It's just your first time. Let me fix you up with a cup of tea and you'll be fine.'

"'Bullshit. That stuff is horrible. Tea ain't gonna do no good. I'm really fucked up. You and your crazy-ass ideas.'

"Frog told me to lighten up and took me into the kitchen, where he made some tea for us. I don't know what kind of chemical reaction it caused, but when I took that cup of tea it was like utopia. It was so damn good. I couldn't believe it. It was wonderful. I imagined this must be like what the older guys go through when they get a heroin high. That's how mean it was. I told Frog I wanted to get some for the next day. It was great.

I remained high all night and most of the next day from just three ounces of the stuff. It was wonderful.

"From then on I started to go to Doc K's almost every day for Tussar syrup. I'd get me three or six ounces, depending on how much money I had, go home, heat up some tea, and mellow out. Man, it was beautiful. Even though I was still doing wine and marijuana, the cough medicine quickly became my favorite. I was over at the drugstore four, sometimes five days a week. I think I became old Doc K's best customer.

"Not too long after that, Hennie, my twenty-year-old cousin, takes me to a drugstore at 18th and York. She leaves me in the front of the store and then goes to the back, where the prescriptions are filled. I guess I wasn't supposed to see this, but I catch this old, gray-haired guy grabbing my cousin's ass. She looks at me, and then the old pharmacist notices I'm there and that I caught him in the act. He got real sheepish. He knew that he got caught doin' something that he shouldn't be doin'.

"My cousin then asked him for $1.50 worth of white bennies and told him, 'Anytime my cousin comes in here for me you give him what he asks

23

for, you hear?' The old guy didn't say a word. He knew he had gotten caught and didn't want any trouble. From then on I was picking up bennies at the drugstore for my cousin and myself. Between the pills, the reefer, tussar, and alcohol, I was a drunken cigar store Indian. I'd be walking the streets and standing on the corner stoned out of my mind. I'd be bug-eyed and swaying like a wobbly pin in a bowling alley. I was so messed up people began calling me 'Bubble-eyed Butch.' They must have thought I was really fucked up and had lost my mind, but I was feeling fine. I was no longer confused, wondering who to listen to or what path to take. The alcohol and drugs were like a confusion reducer and painkiller. I was in my own little world, and for me it was a lot better than the real one."

"Then I got on the big one. Friends introduced me to heroin. I had been doing a lot of reefer, but my friends were older, around seventeen to twenty years old, and they were doing the really hard stuff. They told me, 'Butch, if you really want to get high, try this.' Oh my God. It was the worst experience of my life.

"We were down at a friend's house around 25th and Susquehanna, and I knew they were gonna shoot up. I was very nervous. I had heard about guys dying from overdoses, but I looked up to these guys. They were hip and considered swingers. They were older than me and knew a lot of stuff. I was hanging with them and didn't want them to think I was afraid. I wanted their respect, so I figured I'd give it a shot.

"There was only the three of us in the house at the time, and all we had was a nickel bag. I saw them messing with homemade equipment—a syringe made out of an eyedropper, a baby pacifier, and a needle. It was called a New York works. They did crazy stuff like tear an edge off a dollar bill, wet it, and make a collar that fastened the needle on the eyedropper. Drugs were still rare back then. It was still a hush-hush thing. Not too many people had real syringes. A lot of times you had to make your own equipment.

"They shot me up with a smaller amount than what they gave each other. Oh man, I fell out immediately. I mean passed right out. They slapped me; they punched me. They did everything they could to wake me up. They were getting pretty scared, so they then shot me with some combination of milk and stuff and forced saltwater down my throat to raise my pressure and bring me back. It was their form of street science, but they were scared and racing to counter the effects of the heroin. They knew it was my first time and figured my body wasn't ready for such a jolt. They said I finally came to after about fifteen minutes and vomited for a long time after that.

"I didn't want anything to do with heroin, homemade syringes, or any of that stuff after that first experience. The shit made me sick. About a week later, though, I saw one of the guys, and he says he's got something for me.

"'No way, man,' I told him. 'That junk made me sick. Damn, it nearly killed me.'

"'You got sick because it was your first time,' said Whitey. 'And you didn't coat your stomach.' He says, 'Let me give you a hit of this. You'll love it. But first we're gonna give you some salami and tomato juice. That'll take care of your stomach.'

"My instincts told me no way. That shit had nearly killed me. But once again I let them talk me into it. It always seemed I let the niggers talk me into doing some goddamn crazy thing. I figured I was doing something that was hip. And I looked up to these guys. I wanted to be like them.

"They were right. The second time was totally different. My system welcomed it. I was in heaven. I listened to jazz all day. It was wonderful. I had been turned around. I guess it all started in 1955, when my father died, and then a few years later, when I started drifting away from church and my mother's apron strings. Once I got a taste of drugs, I really turned around."

25

Butch Anthony's gradual slide from alcohol to full-scale heroin addiction accelerated when he started making regular trips up the Jersey turnpike to score a better grade of product in the drug-infested tenements of Harlem. The dangerous Harlem shopping excursions were the culmination of a self-destructive journey that began with those early and presumably innocent sips of beer and wine his siblings offered when his parents weren't home. Little Butch was now in his late teens and had graduated from alcohol, marijuana, codeine, and pills to the next rung on the addiction ladder. He was now seriously hooked on smack. As in the past, older, trusted allies—his homeys—were his tour guides to his sordid life as a heroin addict.

It was in early 1961 that Anthony, his cousin Donald, and two of his "old heads"—Buddy and Vernon—drove up to Manhattan for the first time to cop some heroin. The smack coming out of Harlem was said to be not only the most potent you could purchase, but also considerably cheaper than anything that could be picked up on the streets of Philly. The Harlem outing was an eye-opener for Butch.

Anthony's hometown may have been the nation's third-largest city at the time, but Philly didn't compare to the Big Apple. The heavily trafficked streets and sidewalks, the height and grandeur of the buildings, and the frenetic, pulsating energy of New York made a fitting prelude to his first Harlem buy. The four men drove uptown to a small, nondescript apartment building in the middle of the block near 127th Street and Amsterdam Avenue.

After knocking on the door a couple of times, they finally heard someone bark in a gruff voice, "Who the hell is it? What do you want?"

"It's Buddy from Philly," replied one of Anthony's "old heads."

"Who?"

"Buddy. Buddy from Philly. You know who it is. Don't be fucking with me now."

"Is there anyone with you?"

"Yeah," said Buddy. "A few of my young boys. I'm breaking 'em in."

"I don't know 'em. Who the fuck are they?"

"Listen, nigger," said Buddy, "open the fuckin' door. Everything is cool. I told you who it was."

"I could hear the locks being turned, and then the door opened," recalls Anthony of his first foray to a Harlem drug den. "It was dark as hell in there and really foul smelling. I was able to make out a couple of junkies sitting on a couch. They were nodding off from the heroin. They were barely able to open their eyes, but when they did they greeted Buddy the way junkies do, using slang and slapstick."

"'Hey, what's up, baby? I ain't seen you in ages,' said one of the junkies. 'Are you back here to stay? Man, I miss you. Last time I seen you, you had a bag of some good shit on 117th Street. Those were the days, man.'

"'Nah, I'm not staying. I'm going back to Philly,' said Buddy. 'I only brought my young bloods up here to cop. Where's Diggs?'

"'He's up in the bathroom. He'll be done soon.'

"Buddy said, 'c'mon,' and started walking us through the apartment. The place was a mess and really stunk. You could see no one was taking care of the place. It was a flophouse for junkies. We passed a bedroom, and sitting on a bed and a chair were two junkie sisters nodding off. I later learned they were the house whores.

"We passed a couple other rooms, when Diggs finally emerged from the bathroom. He was a big black guy dressed in long johns, at least the lower half. His hands were big, and he had arms like Popeye's, swollen and covered with abscesses. He looked like a big broiled steak."

Anthony recalls Diggs giving the Philly contingent a warm greeting and embracing Buddy in his muscular, abscess-covered arms. "What's up, my man? Long time no see," said Diggs. "I sure been missing you, baby. What you got for me?"

"It's what you got for me," said Buddy.

"How so, my brother?" asked Diggs.

Buddy leaned close to Diggs and whispered, "I want some stuff. Two-sixteenths of H for my crew."

"Okay, baby," replied Diggs, a big smile spreading across his face. "But you'll have to wait until I get my shot first."

"No problem, man. Take your time," said Buddy.

Diggs pulled out what appeared to be a whole eighth of an ounce of dope and put it in a big Vaseline cap. As usual, a small piece of cotton was placed on top to prevent impurities from being drawn up into the syringe. He poured the entire contents of the bag in the metal cap, and Anthony, as he recalls, "being young and dumb and ignorant of different people's habits," thought there must have been enough dope in the cap to feed everyone in the house.

"I really thought he was gonna turn on everyone in the house. You know, to sample the quality of his stuff. But, to my amazement, this was the guy's shot. And he was probably doing it two or three times a day. I couldn't believe it was one guy's hit.

"After putting water on the dope and cooking it up with a cigarette lighter until the contents dissolved, he took two eyedroppers with a baby's pacifier on the end of it and attached a needle to the small end of the eyedropper and proceeded to draw the dope out of the cooker. One of the sisters came over and tied his arm off with an old stocking, and they started looking for a vein in the midst of all those sores and abscesses. They must have stuck him twenty times before they found a hit where some blood emerged, a sign they had finally found an open vein to inject the drugs. Diggs took an ink pen and circled the area for future reference.

"Ever since my first hit, I'd been concerned about overdosing on the shit. There was always talk on the streets about guys dying from an overdose. It always had me worried, so seeing this crazy guy shooting all this stuff at one time had me convinced he was going down. I figured there's no way this nigger is going to survive this. I'm really looking for this guy to hit the floor, but instead he injects it all without blinking an eye. I said to myself, 'Wow, this motherfucker is really something.' Then, on top of this, he took a second eyedropper full of dope, pulled the eyedropper out while leaving the needle inserted in his arm, and proceeds to inject the second eyedropper of heroin into his system. It was the first time I had ever seen anyone do a piggyback shot.

"I just knew this guy had done it, he was going to die. But instead of crashing to the floor, he begins to sing and dance around the room like he had found his groove. A couple hits and this crazy motherfucker had turned into a black Fred Astair. It was incredible. It wasn't till later that I found out that the New York junkies could shoot ten times more heroin than a guy from Philly or anywhere else. Hell, an eighth used by one New York junkie could be turned into twenty five-dollar shots in Philly.

"After Diggs did his thing, we all shot up there. We all got high. The dope was dynamite. We got in the car and drove around to Braddock's Bar at 127th and 8th Avenue. It was a well-known jazz joint that occasionally attracted some big-name players. It also offered a free drink for every drink you bought. It was our kind of place. Since we were coming up to New York, we were all dressed to kill. I mean, we really looked sharp. I looked so good a girl came up to me at the bar and asked if I was Lee Morgan, the trumpet player from Philly. I said, 'Yeah, baby, but I ain't playing tonight.'

"I don't know if she really confused me with Lee Morgan or was just playin', but she gets a little closer and says to me, 'You sportin'?'

"I thought to myself, 'What the fuck is this? What's this sportin'?' She's eyeing me up and down and I didn't know what to say. I finally turned around to Buddy and asked, 'What's sportin'?'

"'You dumb nigger,' says Buddy, 'that bitch wants to sell you some pussy.'

"I may have seemed like a dumb country boy my first trip up there, but I didn't stay that way. I got the hang of it pretty quick. From then on I'd go up to New York City and cop some good Harlem heroin. Sometimes I'd go up with my crew and sometimes I went up on my own. I'd take the train from Philly to Penn Station and then hop the A train up to Harlem. I'd get off the subway at the first stop after 127th Street and walk to the apartment. I'd knock on the door. Somebody behind the door would say,

'Who's there?' And I'd say, 'Philly,' and they'd let me right in. They got to know me pretty good. I think I became one of their best customers."

Anthony's New York jaunts may have fostered some high times and interesting stories, but his pursuit of the better-grade Harlem heroin was always a problematic venture. Police raids, gangsters ripping off dope dealers and their customers, and the purchase of impure goods were always possibilities. Even the opposite—the acquisition of super-high-grade dope—could result in death. On one New York run, for example, Butch was almost left for dead. He had driven up to Harlem with four friends from the Village—Willie Bo Bo, Pongo, Donald, and Jerry. They all had some spending money and were expecting to score. Butch had raided his brother's wallet—a periodic alternative to stealing on the street—and took the crew to a Harlem contact who had always provided what he needed. The deal was to turn over the money and then wait twenty to thirty minutes for his contact to score the goods and return.

This time it wasn't so simple. Hours went by. Butch and his friends waited in a public park, walked Harlem's bustling streets, and killed time in various bars. They were furious; they had been scammed. Arguing among themselves and fantasizing how they would punish the grifter who had taken them, they tried to figure out what to do next. Finally, while bemoaning their fate on a street corner near Amsterdam Avenue, they spotted their man. Or what was left of him. As Butch recalls, he was doing "deep knee bends, taking three steps and going down. He was fucked up."

Butch was the first to confront the man, yelling, "Give me my shit before I kill you, you son of a bitch." His contact seemed incapable of either talking or standing; he was out on his feet—plastered on dope. Butch and his friends rifled through the man's pockets and took several packages of heroin and what little money he had left. The man put up little resistance but kept muttering, "Don't take the whole shot. Don't take the whole shot. That shit'll kill you."

After quickly claiming the contents of the man's pockets and dumping him in an alley, they hurried back to their car and headed downtown for one of the tunnels to Jersey.

Agitated by the lengthy ordeal and in need of a fix, Butch couldn't wait till he got back home to shoot up. He prepared the cooker and opened a bag of dope while they drove down Manhattan's West Side Highway. Disregarding the disheveled condition of his contact and the advice he had just received, Butch shot a whole bag. He was out cold before the car entered the Holland Tunnel. As his eyes rolled back in his head and he slumped forward, his last words were, "It's bad, man." He didn't regain consciousness until the quintet reached 27th and Westmoreland streets in North Philadelphia.

The trip home, however, was far from uneventful. As they hurtled down the New Jersey Turnpike, Anthony's mates grew concerned and eventually panic stricken; Butch couldn't be revived. The dope was bad. New York heroin was always considered more potent than what could be obtained in Philly, but this was worse than anything they had previously experienced. Whether it was too potent or adulterated with a toxic substance, they suspected Butch had taken a lethal dose of opiate. They slapped him repeatedly, massaged his neck and chest, and threw water in his face, but there was no response. They pulled into a Howard Johnson highway rest stop and purchased milk, salt, and a few other items, and then shot him up with a variety of junkie medicinal elixirs, but nothing worked. He was beyond unconscious. Two of his traveling companions wrote Butch off as another OD casualty and wanted to dump his body in a roadside pine grove. They argued among themselves for some time. No one wanted to bring a dead body back to Philly and be confronted by angry relatives or, worse, police detectives. But his cousin, Donald, insisted that Butch deserved better than being left in a ditch somewhere in New Jersey's Pine Barrens.

When he eventually regained consciousness—albeit with a swollen face and finger marks from the numerous slaps he had received—Butch was seemingly unimpressed by his near-fatal experience. Drugs anesthetized him against the daily struggle and pain of life. He needed them to survive and spent the greater part of each day looking forward to his next joint of Parisian Red or Acapulco Gold, three ounces of cherry codeine, or shot of Harlem heroin. Butch was as capable of getting off drugs as of giving up the air he breathed.

It would take something stronger than a near-fatal overdose to change his ways. Not even the specter of marriage and fatherhood could deter his need for narcotics. In fact, they probably contributed to the emotional turbulence inside his head and the drug habit it fostered.

Butch first met Laura on his way home from the Park Movie Theater at 31st and Diamond streets. He had spent the afternoon with friends at the movies drinking wine and eating hoagies, when he decided he had had enough of the show and left the theater by himself. On the several-block journey home he spotted his future wife.

"She looked like a beautiful China doll," recalls Anthony. "She was a petite, redbone sister with gorgeous dimples and a long graceful neck. I figured she was about three years younger than me, maybe thirteen, but she was the most beautiful thing I had ever seen. Normally I would have been a tongue-tied idiot around such a good-looking female and never opened my mouth for fear of fumbling over my words, but I had been drinking wine all afternoon and was higher than a Georgia pine. Being high on wine, codeine, or marijuana, though, was a different story; it brought the devil out in me. I came out with, 'Oh baby, baby. Come here. I gotta take a good look at you. Aren't you a sweet little thing. What's your name?'

"She was laughing, but still ran in a store at 29th and Susquehanna and asked the proprietor to protect her from this crazy guy that was after her. She eventually came out and nearly broke her neck running away from me. I dreamed about her every night after that.

"Then, about two weeks later, I saw her again. She was walking with my cousin Yogi, and it broke my heart. Yogi was the neighborhood pimp, but I couldn't believe that this beautiful little girl was in his stable.

"'Come here, Butch,' he says, as they approached my house, 'let me introduce you to this sweet little thing. This is Laura.'

"I'm thinking, 'You dirty motherfucker, you broke my heart.' He probably just knew her from the neighborhood, but I still didn't like him being around her. But in reality I can't say a word. I'm sober and near petrified of women, especially good-looking ones like this little Laura. 'Hello, pleased to meet you,' is all I can get out of my mouth."

Though Laura may have wondered if this well-behaved, reticent young man was the same Butch Anthony who had so boldly approached her on the street that day, she was still taken by him. When in public and not under the influence of pills, reefer, or Tussar syrup, Butch was "mild, gentle, and considerate," and those tender, passive qualities appealed to Laura. In the following weeks they spied each other on a playground or at a mutual friend's house and spent a good share of their time surreptitiously glancing at each other. Butch could be playing basketball and Laura participating in a nearby track meet, but their athletic endeavors were clearly secondary to their growing interest in each other.

Before long, Laura and Butch were a loving couple. Surprisingly, she wasn't too disturbed by Butch's attraction to drugs. She relished those times when he was his natural, sweet self and appreciated his periodic visits to her home, a daunting trek across arbitrary neighborhood boundaries that could easily get one killed. Their love affair endured for a year or more, and then hit a critical juncture: Laura told him she was pregnant. She wanted to get married, but Butch resisted.

"Why don't you want to marry me?" asked Laura. "I know you love me."

"You know what I do," argued Butch, referring to his drug use. "What kind of a husband do you think I would make? Sometimes I'm so high I can't even function. How would I support you and the baby? I'm sick. I'll ruin your life."

Laura said she didn't care. She'd help him kick his addiction. She said she loved him and wanted to marry him, but Butch could see no good coming from the union. In addition to his drug use, he was preoccupied by the notion that every male in the Village was after her. She was a natural beauty, and every guy in North Philly was always coming on to her, sometimes even in his presence. She didn't encourage the catcalls, whistles, and comments, but when he was with her Butch was always anticipating a fight with one of her many admirers. It put him on edge. Their "come-on" lines to her made him furious.

"I was madly in love with her," says Butch, "but I didn't trust her. Every guy in the neighborhood wanted her. I was crazy in love, but the situation drove me nuts."

And now she was carrying his child. Though they debated the options her pregnancy presented, Laura couldn't talk Butch into marriage. Finally she said, "All right, I'll get rid of it."

Preoccupied by the stressful situation, Butch was now ingesting three times the number of pills he had previously been consuming. When not downing a variety of pinks and whites, he inquired around as to how such a deed should be done. He was offered a variety of "down-home" and "back-alley" abortion remedies, but finally settled on something that seemed relatively simple—Laura plopping herself down in a tub full of mustard powder and hot water. He was assured that the odd but simple recipe would do the trick. Fortunately, one of Butch's sisters caught the guilty-looking pair on a street corner with the newly purchased bag of mustard seed powder and pressed them for an explanation.

"Where are you two going?" asked Peasie. "What do you have in that bag?"

Neither teenager spoke up.

"You heard me," said Peasie. "What are you two up to?"

"I'm pregnant," Laura replied timidly. "We're gonna get rid of the baby."

"Are you out of your fucking mind?" screamed Butch's sister. "Are you crazy? Throw that fucking shit down the sewer. Forget that dumb shit. You're not getting rid of no baby."

It was November 1961, a time when the phrase "shotgun marriage" was still in use, and the Anthony family had no intention of letting its youngest member slide; he wouldn't be absolved of his familial responsibility.

"You no-good nigger," screamed Butch's mother on hearing the bad news. "You got that young girl pregnant. What are you gonna do now?"

"Don't worry," replied Butch. "I'm gonna pay the bills."

"No," shouted Mrs. Anthony. "You're gonna marry that girl. You come from a good family, a religious family. You're gonna make sure that child has a name."

By the time the wedding was held, on November 11, 1961, at the Anthony residence on 27th Street, Edward "Butch" Anthony was a walking pharmacy. As he recalls, he was "so fucked up on drugs," thanks to the conflagration of opposing pressures surrounding the marriage, it would take him "weeks to come down to earth."

Paralyzed with fear that it wasn't marriage but "judgment day" he was facing, and pulverized by an assortment of uppers and downers, Butch was discovered in bed just hours before the service by his older brothers Joe and Wilbert. He was frozen with fear, smelled awful, and hadn't changed his clothes in days.

"Listen, nigger," yelled his intimidating brother, Joe, "if you think you're gonna embarrass the family with this act, you're crazy. You got your sorry ass in this mess. Now you're gonna be a man and face the consequences."

Joe and Wilbert dragged Butch out of bed, threw him in the bathtub, and washed him thoroughly. Though they clothed him and then delivered him to the Reverend David DeBrady, who was waiting with the rest of the wedding party in the living room, Butch was firmly planted in another world.

For the drug-sated groom, this was not a wedding ceremony but the "end of the world." "Everything was about dying," recalls Butch. "The reverend looked like the executioner, and people were walking through walls like ghosts. I really thought my mother and the others were trying to kill me."

"Bubble-Eyed Butch"

Standing as stiff as a board, his bubble-eyed Butch facial expression even more pronounced than usual, the groom was in full delusional flight. When he heard the words, "Will you take this woman," he swore that Reverend DeBrady's eyes were on fire, horns protruding from his head, and smoke emanating from his fingertips. Even his beloved Laura was a vision of devilish images. "I was expecting the whole world would end," he recalls.

When it was time to place the ring on her finger, he was incapable of the simple task and had to have assistance holding the ring. Laura slipped her finger through the ring while Butch stood mesmerized with fear. Just as they were pronounced man and wife and Laura raised her veil to kiss her husband, she broke into tears. Seeing her husband's actual condition was just too disturbing; she nearly fled the house without him.

The wedding over, Laura stood on the corner, a tattered suitcase by her side. Her husband, however, refused to leave the house. Not until his mother shoved him out the door and locked it behind him did he join his bride on the sidewalk. It is difficult to imagine a marriage getting off to a worse start.

The newlyweds went to live with one of Butch's aunts, who lived around the corner at 26th and Dauphin streets. Without the benefit of a honeymoon or any viable prospects to speak of, the couple settled down as much as they could, considering Butch's bewildered mental state—he was practically catatonic. He remained in bed twenty-four hours a day, uncommunicative, the bubble-eyed Butch stare planted squarely on his face. Fearful and exasperated, Laura could only wonder what was going through her husband's head.

"I was seeing monsters," recalls Butch of those terrible days. "I saw people walking through walls, people on TV talking to me and saying my name, and smoke rising from the eyes and ears of everybody I came in contact with. There were times I thought I was Jesus and God was talking to me. I was completely paranoid and delusional. Man, it was terrible."

Increasingly worried about her husband's bizarre behavior, a distraught Laura went to see her mother-in-law for advice. Butch's mother wasted little time in addressing the situation. "Look at you," she shouted at the bedside of her son. "Staring in space like a goddamn zombie. You're a mess. You're a disgrace. Get out of that bed. I'm taking you to a doctor."

Mrs. Anthony dragged her youngest and by far most problematic child over to Dr. Lindenbaum's office at 26th and York. After talking to both mother and son and examining Butch thoroughly, the doctor gave them

his assessment. Butch had suffered a nervous breakdown due to a combination of competing social pressures and overdosing on amphetamine and
Benzedrine pills. By imbibing more than a dozen pills a day since he had
learned of Laura's pregnancy, he had become paranoid and delusional. The
doctor gave him an injection and prescribed medication and a therapeutic
regimen of activities that resulted in Butch's condition gradually improving.
Within three weeks, Laura had her Butch back.

Though Butch's mental state returned to normal, the couple's economic
and marital prospects remained very shaky. Butch had dropped out of
Thomas Edison High School the year before. Education wasn't his thing;
the only course he excelled at was an upholstery shop class. No matter, he
rationalized, he'd join the Marines and serve in the military like his older
brothers had. Unfortunately, his educational deficiencies came back to
haunt him. He failed the entrance test by two points.

Without a high school diploma and lacking ambition, Butch took a series
of menial, low-paying jobs. He was a stock boy at Jeff's Grocery and did
some heavy lifting at the Corbin Brothers pipe-fitting plant at 25th and York.
Neither job put him and Laura on easy street. His best job, money-wise, was
at Connolly Containers in North Philadelphia.

"At sixteen I got the job at Crown, Cork & Seal at 'G' and Erie. I was
pretty young, but they were hiring college kids for the summer, so I didn't
look too much out of place. I ran a slither machine that chopped the metal
up in sections that were then molded into soda cans. It was hard work,
but I was making $9 an hour, and that was way above minimum wage.
And that was back then. The money allowed me to make regular runs up
to New York. I had the job for about a year and a half, and then I got fired
for using drugs."

The loss of steady legal income forced Butch to ramp up his illicit hustles.
Working with a coterie of similarly desperate friends from the Village,
Butch started spending more and more time in other people's homes.
Working in both the neighborhood and more upscale environs, Butch and
his friends were breaking into private residences several times a week.
Generally, they targeted number writers, storeowners, and businessmen
who they knew had money. When a phone call or knock at the door went
unanswered, they'd break a window and enter the residence.

"My heart be pounding like a motherfucker," Butch recalls of his break-ins.
"You had to have heart or you couldn't do that line of work."

Televisions, electrical appliances, and clothing were all good to go. Then a brief negotiation with a fence or an impromptu neighborhood "red tag sale," and Butch had what he needed—money for drugs. Butch's second-story work should not be confused with more successful and professional Philadelphia burglary rings such as Kensington's K & A Gang.[1] Butch and his crewmates were relative novices and were usually lucky to clear $100 per man a night. About the only similarity in their operations is that both groups rejected violence and never carried weapons while on a job. As Butch says, "We weren't out to hurt anybody, we just wanted to make some money to get drugs. We never used a gun. There were never any stickups. I could never do anything physical that would hurt somebody. It was against my morals."

In addition to burglary, Butch fed his habit through an array of illegal gambits that included boosting anything he could get his hands on. Any item of value that wasn't nailed down, from clothing to food products, was fair game. Butch and his fellow junkies, for example, scammed every supermarket in the city. They'd each wear a button-down sweater and a sturdy belt around the waist that could be fastened as tightly as necessary, depending upon the assortment of goods surreptitiously stashed inside the garment. A large, roomy overcoat was worn on top to cover any pur-loined goods protruding from the sweater. Butch claims that six to eight good-sized steaks could be hidden in such a fashion.

Their system was simple. They'd enter a supermarket, grab a pushcart, and drop an assortment of items into their basket. The real action, how-ever, started when they entered the meat aisle. Butch and an accomplice would face each other, thereby observing whether anyone was watching them, and, when the opportunity presented itself, start shoving beef inside their sweaters. Six good-sized steaks, three on each side of their fastened sweaters, was the typical haul.

Along with accomplices to gather goods and distract shop owners, ten dollars a man to hire a driver to chauffer them around to various stores, and the use of additional ploys, such as pinning closed the sleeves of jackets to conceal shoplifted items and collecting discarded receipts from supermarket floors, Butch and his friends had quite a hustle going. Several trips a day to a Penn Fruit on North Broad Street or an Acme supermarket on City Line Avenue that catered to a more upscale clientele paid off with a wide selection of top-shelf provisions. Back in the hood, Butch and his accomplices became well-known wholesalers who offered steep discounts to friends and neighbors looking for a good deal.

"We took the meat and groceries to houses throughout the neighborhood," says Butch, "and sold them for a third or more off the sticker price. A $60 pack of meat would sell for $40, and they'd be pretty good cuts of beef. Folks loved getting prime cuts of filet mignon and sirloin steak that local groceries in the Village never carried and that they couldn't afford even if they did. We became so well known in the community that when we'd knock on a door little kids inside would see us and call out to their mothers, 'Hey mom, the meat man is here.'"

Butch's street hustles suddenly turned sour when he was pinched for selling marijuana in 1963. Duped by a friend into selling some reefer to a black undercover cop on Diamond Street, Butch spent several hours at the police station at 22nd and Hunting Park Avenue before being transferred to Moyamensing Prison in South Philadelphia. Moyamensing, better known as "Moko" to the local criminal element, was an aging relic from the 1830s, with wooden floors, austere cell blocks, and unusual Egyptian architectural appointments, that was on the verge of being closed and decommissioned. Butch's first time in a prison would be a chilling experience he wouldn't soon forget.

"Man," says Butch, "it was like a house of horrors. That joint was rough. It was a real dark, primitive, claustrophobic place and reminded me of something out of the old cowboy pictures. There were three to a cell, the floors were made of wooden planks, big pots were used to hold beverages in the mess hall, and there were guys always boxing in this little exercise yard that was no bigger than a basketball court. I was only twenty, and one of the youngest ones in there. All the tough guys from my neighborhood seemed to be there. The place was dangerous; I never wanted to go out of my cell for fear I'd end up in a fight, or worse.

"I was hearing all these stories about foot-long rats in the prison's sewer system, different gangs that ran the blocks, and young boys getting raped. Hearing about things like 'shit shanks,' where guys got their dicks infected from fucking guys up the ass and then needing doctors to massage their prostate and bang their dicks with a hammer to knock the shit out, scared the hell out of me. That place was mean. I wanted to scream out, 'get me out of this fucking place.'"

Butch got his wish about a month and a half later, when he was transferred to another ancient city jail—Holmesburg. He recognized fairly quickly, however, that the trip to the larger jail in Northeast Philadelphia was not a step up. "The Burg," as it was informally known, was a fearsome walled facility dating back to the 1890s with its own formidable history, which included everything from flying squads of prison toughs who flogged new inmates at the behest of the warden, to a particularly savage punishment unit called the "Klondike," where malcontents were given the heat treatment, which on one occasion resulted in the infamous "Bake Oven Deaths."[2]

Though he was unfamiliar with the institution's ominous history, Butch was impressed with what he saw going on around him. "There were guys in there doing life bits and twenty- to forty-year sentences. I mean, some real bad fucking dudes were in there. It sounded and looked like a state joint. I sure as hell didn't think I belonged there."

Fortunately, Butch caught a break when he finally went to court on the sales charge after being locked up in Holmesburg for nearly two months. Though the judge hit Butch with two separate eleven-and-a-half- to twenty-three-month sentences, he ended up sentencing him to time served. Butch was ecstatic. He'd be on parole for some time, but he was a free man. Never a particularly good student, however, the lessons he learned from the arrest and his internment at dismal and dangerous places like Moko and the Burg did not stick. Butch went back to his old ways, including his abiding attraction to narcotics. "I was fucking up," says Butch. "I couldn't help myself." Within months he was back in jail again. Picked up for shoplifting clothes at Jerry's Corner, a neighborhood haberdasher, his parole was revoked and he was incarcerated in the city's newest prison, the Detention Center. Butch would now have to do his original twenty-three-month sentence.

Both he and the other inmates he associated with knew he didn't belong there. Though he tried to pass as a streetwise tough guy from the Village who could more than hold his own with the other menacing brothers prowling the institution's dormitories and cell blocks, his gentle, sensitive nature gave him away. "Hey man," he was often asked, "what the hell are you doing in here?"

His meager efforts to blend in at DC were rudely interrupted when he was suddenly transferred to Holmesburg in early 1964. He now faced the prospect of doing at least two years in the toughest jail in the city. No more relaxed dormitory settings in a newly constructed facility, no more "close-watch" quarantine periods. He'd now be out in population and housed on leaky and dilapidated cell blocks with some of the "scariest dudes" on the East Coast. But in addition to being confined behind bars and separated from family and friends, Edward "Butch" Anthony would soon discover something else—that he had been sentenced to science, as well.

39

"Don't Serve Time; Let Time Serve You"

"Man, when I walked into the center of Holmesburg that first time, it scared the hell out of me. When I saw all those guys patched up, wrapped up, bandages and gauze pads all the hell over them, I said to myself, 'Oh my God. What the hell did I walk into? These muthafuckers are killing each other in here.' I thought it was World War III.

"I really did. I thought these muthafuckers are carving and stabbing the hell out of each other. It was one violent goddamn joint. Holmesburg had the worst, most treacherous dudes in the world in there. Nasty, mean, muscle-bound killers all covered in medical tape and hospital dressing. It was on their arms, their legs, their backs, their heads. 'Man,' I said to myself, 'they're killing each other in here. I sure as hell don't wanna be in here. I want my mother.'

"I was a young dude and pretty sensitive. It was almost too much for me to handle. I had heard the stories about Holmesburg, but seeing it for real had me fucked up. I'm telling you, I was scared to death."

4

Eddie Anthony's frightened reaction to seeing the University of Pennsylvania's human research program at Holmesburg Prison wasn't that unusual for someone getting his first glimpse of a large-scale clinical trial—especially one operating within the claustrophobia-inducing walls of a prison. The specter of human research on a grand scale at a maximum-security facility could be literally breathtaking, not to mention chilling, particularly for someone unfamiliar with the primitive atmosphere so common to correctional institutions. Penal institutions have an atavistic air about them that naturally fosters violent, menacing images. Combine that with scores of inmates adorned in medical dressing, and one's fears can easily become apocalyptic.

Anthony had been in the jail for ten days, but he was being held on C block, a quarantine unit for new arrivals. Freedom was restricted and movement off the block was prohibited. Signs of human research at the facility were practically nonexistent from Anthony's limited vantage point. The only hint of such a program came, curiously enough, from the less threatening and friendlier members of the prison's social service department.

"We were locked down on the block for almost two weeks. We rarely left our cells, and that was only to get physical exams for any diseases or medical conditions we might be bringing into the jail. They were checking for things like syphilis and TB. One of the social workers came around during these orientation briefings to inform us what was expected of us and gave us the handbook of institutional infractions that contained the rules and regulations of the jail. He went through all the disciplinary policies and what actions would be taken against anyone who disobeyed them. He then started to go into all the programs the jail offered, such as sports and educational programs.

"At the end of it all he said something that really caught my attention. He said while we were locked up we should try and get our act together. 'Don't serve time,' he said. 'Let time serve you. Get in the programs and try to become a trustee.' He then jumped right into the testing program. He said, 'For inmates with low bails or those that need money, we have the University of Pennsylvania research program.' He said the tests the doctors were doing were safe and guys could earn some money, money that we could send home to our families or use to purchase things in the commissary like ice cream, potato chips, candy, and personal grooming items.

"It sounded pretty good to me, but I wasn't really sure what he was talking about. I didn't really know anything about the testing going on, but I got the idea it would allow me to be a little more independent. I wouldn't have to depend on loan sharks for money or be foolin' around with any asshole bandits. I really paid attention to the presentation when they started talkin' about money. My family hadn't come up to see me since I was arrested. They took a hard line. All they said was, 'You made your bed, now lay down in it.'

"It was pretty clear I wouldn't be getting any financial help from them. My family cut me loose. I didn't really understand what all the testing was about, but if I could make some money from it, maybe it was a good thing."

The social workers knew equally little about the research that was under way, but it didn't stop them from encouraging the inmate population to participate in the program. In fact, few Holmesburg staff members had any inkling of what the research was about. As usual, if the penal administrators at the top of the custody food chain gave the human research program the "Good Housekeeping Seal of Approval," then it was beyond criticism. No one questioned the research program's utility, legitimacy, or ethics, especially not the overworked and understaffed prison social workers. "We only knew what we were told," says Tom Shouler, a social worker who worked at the jail for several decades. "It was the University of Pennsylvania program to test new cosmetics and perfumes. We never knew any more than that."[1]

Adds Scott Willson, one of Shouler's colleagues, "Nobody really investigated what the tests were about. The medical personnel walked around in white coats and looked very official and authoritative."[2] It didn't take long for the university testing program to fill a key niche in the prison culture.

"If somebody didn't have money for commissary and wasn't on the list for a job, the social worker would say, 'You can go to the U of P testing operation,'" says Priscilla Becroft, another social worker. "The medical program was thought to be benign at the time."[3]

Anthony got his first serious glimpse of the research program when he and a dozen or so other inmates were taken off the quarantine block and shipped to their new housing assignments. Anthony was assigned to G block, his new home in general population. He had to cross "center" to get there, a large piece of circular real estate that was actually a huge nineteenth-century rotunda-like structure that formed the hub or axis of the ten cell blocks that made up the jail. For many inmates, it was like walking into Times Square after spending the winter in a darkened cave. Newcomers considered it a full frontal assault on the senses. Seeing scores of hardened, captive men—many of them in various stages of medical care and rehabilitation—was nothing short of stunning.

"One morning the guards came on the block, and we were each given a box of sheets, pillow cases, socks, soap, toothbrush, toothpaste, and one letterhead. They were shipping us to our new housing areas. When they took us off the quarantine unit and marched us through center, I got a chill up my spine. The whistles, catcalls, and the sight of all these men with cups and bandages on their heads and arms—man, it didn't take

43

long to know this was a real violent place. My eyes nearly exploded out of my head. I couldn't get over how many men looked like they had been in the fight of their lives.

"I was taken to G block and placed in a cell with two other dudes. I recognized one from the street, but I wouldn't call him a friend. They were completely crazy. All they did was fight. All day and all night they're in their underwear with bandanas around their heads, boxing. And I don't mean tapping each other; they were pounding each other. I thought, 'Oh my god, I'm gonna get killed with these guys. They're gonna want me to box, too, and I'm gonna end up looking like raw hamburger.' I mean, they were a couple of nuts, and I didn't know how I was gonna survive in there. I knew enough to know you gotta handle yourself in a certain way and stay outta other people's business, but whatta you do when you're locked up with two fight machines? I was getting real familiar with why guys were so bandaged up in Holmesburg.

"The next morning, as we're taken off the block to go to soup alley and breakfast, I run into Youngie [Edward Young], an old head from my neighborhood who's also locked on G block. Youngie's a tough dude and also pretty smart. I tell him what's going on in my cell and that I think I'm gonna have a problem. He tells me to stay cool, but I'm still wondering how I'm gonna survive this place.

"Later that morning the guard comes to my cell and calls me out in the corridor. I'm thinking, 'What now?' But it was only the guard moving me to the rear of the cell block, to 784 cell. Youngie had put a good word in for me with the guards and got me moved to their crib. He was in a cell with another guy from the neighborhood, Ruben Hayes. Both Youngie and Ruben were older and more experienced than me. I was just twenty years old and new to it all, but they were in their thirties and forties and had been around. People respected them. Ruben had fought in the ring and made a rep for himself, and Youngie could handle himself as well, but it was more through the use of his brain than his muscle. He knew how to talk and get over on people. I knew they'd watch my back in there.

"All that first day and night, Youngie and Ruben were mentoring me on the ins and outs of the jail. I could tell they knew what they were talking about because of the way guys talked to them. And their cell was like a minicommissary. The cell was filled with cigarettes, candy bars, ice cream, movie tickets, and cosmetics. Most guys didn't have anything, but Youngie and Ruben were like a grocery store. They were doing pretty good.

"They told me who to stay away from and who not to fuck with. They told me not to mess with the Black Muslims and other guys who would only end up getting me in trouble. They told me stories about all the sex that was going down in the jail, how asshole bandits would get over on you, the blanket parties that you had to watch out for, and what not to get involved with. They were really counseling me on how to survive in the joint.

"Later that first night, we hear a couple guys pushing a cart by the cell. They were giving out medication and signing guys up for tests. Youngie goes over to the door and says, 'Hey Moose, what you got today?'

"This big black guy pushing the cart replies, 'I got this test and this test and this test.'

"When he mentions a Johnson & Johnson bubble bath test, Youngie says, 'That sounds good. I got a homey with me who could use some money, but he don't wanna get hurt. You sure this bubble bath test is all right?' Moose said it was the safest one he had, and Youngie wrote my name down on the clipboard holding the names of volunteers for the U of P testing program.

"Youngie told me the tests were one of the few ways to make money in jail. I told him they scared the hell out of me. Guys looked all fucked up with these bandages, adhesive tape, and cups all the hell over them. I wasn't sure if I wanted any part of it. Youngie said, 'You got somebody sending you money? Somebody gonna be helping you out while you're in here? You better settle down and get on the tests. Start making some money or you're gonna have a rough time in here.'

"I knew what he was talking about. My family had disowned me. They weren't sending anything; they weren't visiting me. I knew if I was gonna make it on my own, this would have to be one of the ways. Youngie said he had checked the thing out and I wouldn't be hurt. This was one of the best tests you could be on, a bubble bath test. I was listening to what he was saying and kept on thinking about what the social worker had said at orientation. 'Don't serve time. Let time serve you.' I told Youngie, okay, I'd do it, and the next morning they called me down to H block."

Butch Anthony's decision to become a human guinea pig wasn't as unusual as one might think. The practice of giving up one's blood or body to authoritative white men cloaked in crisp white smocks with the letters M.D. after their names had been going on for years. Jails and prisons from Maine to California were filled with a motley collection of ruthless murderers, gutsy bank robbers, cunning burglars, slick con men, and just ordinary down-and-out drunks and vagrants who—in a moment of weakness or despera-tion—contemplated becoming grist for the research mill. For generations, hundreds—probably thousands—of incarcerated Americans across the country had been offering their bodies to science.

From early in the twentieth century, prisoners were sought by medical researchers as cheap and available test subjects. Institutions holding vulnerable populations such as orphans, retarded children, and the aged and infirm were also favorite sites for human experimentation. By the mid-1960s, however, when Butch Anthony apprehensively walked onto H block at Holmesburg, prisoners had become not only a staple of Amer-ican research but the guinea pigs of choice for medical and pharmaceuti-cal investigators.[4]

The tradition of subjecting the convicted to imprisonment—and occa-sionally to science as well—was well established. Almost a hundred years ago, for example, Mississippi prisoners played a vital role in the discovery of the cause and treatment of pellagra, a deadly disease that ravaged poor communities across the nation.[5] Particularly insidious in the Deep South, pellagra inspired fears of epidemic in Georgia, Alabama, and Florida, and was associated with "the four D's": dermatitis, diarrhea, dementia, and death. Physicians at the time blamed everything from poor sanitary habits to flawed hereditary traits for the disease, without making a noticeable dent in either the morbidity or the mortality rates. Each year thousands of people contracted pellagra, with its distinctive signature—"the red flame"—a reddening of both hands and feet and an ugly skin rash across the face. Ten percent of those struck by the disease ended up not only disfigured and shunned but dead as well. In Missis-sippi alone there were sixteen thousand new cases in 1915 and more than fifteen hundred deaths. Pellagra had become a deadly affliction in many southern states, inspiring the same kind of fear and loathing leprosy or the plague must have instilled in the Middle Ages.

Fortunately, Joseph Goldberger, a physician with the U.S. Public Health Service, had been watching the annual loss of life with interest from afar, and he developed a theory about the root cause of pellagra. He contacted Governor Earl Brewer of Mississippi and told him he might be able to assist in the fight against pellagra, but he'd need the governor's coopera-tion. His request was simple: he'd need test subjects—preferably white males—to experiment on.

With little to lose, Brewer complied by turning the Rankin Prison Farm over to the northern public health official. To encourage prisoner participation and assuage fears, the governor offered the institution's residents a deal—inmate volunteers would receive a pardon and be set free if they survived Goldberger's experiments. The chance to walk out of Rankin—a typically brutal southern work farm where death rarely took a holiday—was enormously enticing. The promise of a gubernatorial pardon inspired scores to volunteer, but Goldberger said a dozen inmates would be sufficient for his purposes.

Relocated to the prison hospital, the test subjects—at least half were serving life terms for murder—continued their regular prison routine, ate the normal prison fare, and were treated like the farm's other oppressed inhabitants. Gradually, however, Dr. Goldberger started to tinker with their meals. He didn't starve them—they had plenty to eat—but he did remove certain items from their plates. Initially there was little change, but as his dietary meddling progressed the men started to complain; they were increasingly lethargic, unable to complete their institutional chores, and beginning to carp about physical aches and pains in their backs, legs, and joints.

Goldberger was encouraged by the results and further altered the men's dietary intake. Soon the test subjects were sick of the steady diet of cornbread, mush, collard greens, sweet potatoes, grits, and rice, as well as the dizziness, diarrhea, and aches and pains with which they were now plagued. The inmates wanted out and pled to be returned to the general prison population, but Goldberger refused. They had volunteered; they'd have to stay the course.

Finally, in mid-September, after eight months of dietary experimentation, the prisoners started to show the first skin lesions on their hands, faces, and scrotums. By the end of the month all twelve men, now almost totally incapacitated, bore the embarrassing red rash—the much-feared mark of pellagra.

Dr. Goldberger had correctly theorized that pellagra was due to the South's regional diet of fatback, meal, and molasses, which supplied calories but not the necessary protein for a healthy diet. Milk, vegetables, and fresh meat, Goldberger argued, would go a long way in eradicating the scourge of pellagra.

An appreciative Governor Brewer honored his agreement and set the ailing test subjects free. As one relieved volunteer said, "I have been through a thousand hells," adding that he would often have welcomed a bullet if only he could be done with the test. Others said they would have welcomed a "lifetime of hard labor" rather than go through such "a hellish experiment" again. When offered free medical attention until they were fully recovered, the men reacted as if sentenced to death and ran off "like a lot of scared rabbits"—a telling response that would be played out repeatedly by incarcerated test subjects over the next century. Doctors were no longer equated with relief but much the reverse.

Goldberger's scientific triumph not only solved the riddle of a deadly disease, it also underscored the vast potential of prison inmates as medical guinea pigs. For the next two decades, however, American prisons were used as human research centers only sporadically. That's not to say that some fairly bizarre medical experiments didn't still take place behind prison walls. From 1918 to 1922, for instance, Dr. L. L. Stanley performed hundreds of bizarre testicular transplants at San Quentin Penitentiary in California.[6] Convinced that aged and ill men could be reinvigorated and their sexual potency restored through such surgical procedures, he even implanted the testicular matter of rams, goats, and boars in dozens of imprisoned Californians. Dedicated to "pursuing the truth, wherever it may lead," Stanley was sure his operations were "practically painless" and promoted "bodily well-being."

There is no record of just how the inmate test subjects felt about such unusual and invasive goings-on, but Stanley certainly appreciated that his work "could be carried out in a prison, for in such a place all men are treated alike, and live under the same conditions of food, work, and general surroundings." Stanley wasn't the only researcher to find such characteristics terribly appealing, but the field was still relatively small, and the few doctors performing penal studies were generally solitary figures pursuing scientific advancement and personal glory.

The inmates—presuming they had a choice—had their own vision: freedom. A pattern was emerging: the possibility of a pardon for volunteering to be a test subject. Although the prospect of becoming a human guinea pig no doubt chilled the spines of most prison inmates, there were always plenty of others who were willing to roll the dice. Many years behind bars has a way of doing that to a person. Generally poor, uneducated, and prone to risky behavior, inmates, especially those facing long prison terms, sometimes found the offer of a pardon irresistible.

Carl Erickson and Mike Schmidt, for example, two Colorado cons serving long sentences for murder and rape, volunteered to become human guinea pigs in a 1934 tuberculosis study at Denver's National Jewish Hospital.[7] Though concerned—Schmidt said, "I don't exactly relish the idea of making an experiment of myself"—the men were willing to gamble their health in a high-stakes game that could win them a gubernatorial pardon and their freedom. The discomfiting specter of doing a life sentence behind bars could easily make such gambles attractive.

It was the onset of World War II, however, that really transformed the practice of using prison inmates as test subjects into a big business. Combat was taking a drastic toll on American fighting men, but so was disease. In the South Pacific especially, soldiers involved in jungle warfare were as likely to be felled by Anopheles mosquitoes as they were by enemy bullets. In order to fight the staggering human loss to diseases such as malaria, typhus, and dysentery, the Roosevelt administration poured millions of dollars into the coffers of hospitals, colleges, and corporate institutions. While the government funds mobilized resources, the establishment of research sites capable of testing dozens of subjects at a time became a significant hurdle. Where to find an unlimited supply of test subjects? The answer: behind bars.

In the war on malaria, research programs were established at four prisons, the largest one at Atlanta Federal Penitentiary and Stateville Prison in Illinois.[8] Hundreds of prisoners volunteered—their contribution to the war effort—and quickly found themselves being bitten by hungry mosquitoes in the prison hospital, all under the fascinated eye of medical researchers. Raging fever, nausea, vomiting, blackouts, and an endless string of medicinal potions would quickly follow.

So taken by the selfless act was *Life* magazine that its reporters captured the human drama on film and said proudly of the Stateville malaria volunteers, "These one-time enemies of society appreciate to the fullest extent just how completely this is everybody's war."[9]

Though the hyperbole may have been justified, some guinea pigs were no doubt praying for something more tangible—a pardon. After the war, their prayers were answered. Governor Adlai Stevenson pardoned more than two-thirds of the 432 prisoners who had participated in the studies, including twenty-four murderers and one rapist.

Of course, there were additional reasons to volunteer as a test subject. The prospect of getting off a loud, dangerous cell block and into a relatively cozy hospital ward with better food seduced some men, while others used the opportunity to flaunt their manliness. Monetary rewards could always produce volunteers, but freedom remained the coin of the realm when it came to incentives.

The act of self-sacrifice for the good of science won public support, as well. Nathan Leopold, of Leopold and Loeb infamy, for example, won a pardon in the late 1950s after penning his best-selling autobiography, *Life Plus 99 Years,* thereby shortening his life-plus sentence considerably. Several chapters of his book were devoted to the Stateville malaria tests and helped cement in readers' minds Leopold's role as a patriotic test subject serving his country.

The war years sparked a variety of research projects behind prison walls that ran the gamut, from exotic blood tests and new techniques for skin grafting to treatments for sexually transmitted diseases. These were no longer solitary ventures by visionary, albeit sometimes wacky, physicians. They were now large, well-funded, adequately staffed programs, orchestrated by accomplished researchers aligned with major concerns—hospitals, universities, and pharmaceutical companies. Human research in prisons had arrived, but would the practice continue once the war was over?

It didn't take long for the answer to come in. Postwar medical research behind bars not only continued, it took off. The war against Germany and Japan had evolved seamlessly into the war against disease. Government monies appropriated for science and investigational studies climbed annually, and researchers used prisoners for everything from flash burn studies to polio and cancer experiments. All of this, interestingly enough, in the aftermath of the Nuremberg Code—the much-esteemed ten-point document designed to ensure that the horrors of Nazi medicine would never again be visited on human subjects, especially incarcerated test subjects.

The American medical community, however, pled ignorance or professed the belief that the code was crafted only for Nazi physicians. Physicians in America desired an unfettered research landscape, one that called for a minimalist approach to the conduct of medicine and scientific research. Self-interest had clearly trumped professional ethics. As medical historian David Rothman has written, "the utilitarian ethic" prevalent at the time ushered in the "gilded age of research."[10]

Suddenly, institutions holding large numbers of vulnerable people— orphans, the mentally challenged, the destitute, the imprisoned—became valuable commodities. The raw material inside—cut off from family and friends as well as the general public—could be used as desired. This went double for those inside thirty-five-foot prison walls. Physicians with access to penal institutions quickly learned that they could greatly enhance their income by hosting clinical trials for the drug industry, and serious medical researchers were equally quick to grasp the advantages of using a stable population that was locked down and out of public view.

Some doctors did so well that they gave up their private practices in the free world to coordinate prison research full time. One ambitious medical entrepreneur established prison research projects in three separate states and maximized his profits—as many other cost-conscious researchers did—by hiring inmates instead of doctors and nurses to conduct the experiments.[11] Considerable money could be saved in this manner, although the inmate test subjects who had dirty needles used on them, or the incorrect blood type intravenously injected into them, may be excused for being less than enthusiastic about the practice.

Despite such sins—and the potentially deadly repercussions—federal, state, and local prisons threw open their doors to researchers. At least half the states in the Union eventually had a prison or two performing human experiments. Some, like Pennsylvania along "pharmaceutical valley," had more than half a dozen penal institutions hosting human drug trials. Viral hepatitis studies at Clinton Farms in New Jersey, polio field trials and live cancer cell injections in Ohio, mind-control experiments in Iowa, syphilis and amoebic dysentery studies in Seagoville, Texas, and testicular irradiation experiments in Oregon and Washington State are just a few of the research projects that found a home in American prisons.[12]

The Ohio cancer experiments were coordinated by Chester M. Southam, an up-and-coming immunologist based at Manhattan's Sloan-Kettering Institute who was eager to "discover the secret of how healthy human bodies fight the invasion of malignant cells."[13] Prisoners, he said, were "a stable group of people" whose situation contributed to "assurance of continuity" in the scientific process, a clear advantage over doing research on those in the free world, who were "more difficult to work with" because of their "unrestrained and unrestricted" status. When asked about the prospect of test subjects contracting the dreaded disease, Dr. Southam replied that he was fairly certain the immune systems of inmate test subjects would repel the disease. However, if the cancer cells did multiply and spread, he argued, "they could be removed quickly by surgery." As to the Nuremberg Code passed just a decade earlier, Southam replied, "I was unaware of the Nuremberg Code and its code of conduct."[14]

The freewheeling, no-holds-barred atmosphere of these medical studies on prisoners made it a glorious time to do human research. As one intrepid practitioner commented, "I began to go to the prison regularly, although I had no authorization. It was years before the authorities knew that I was conducting various studies on prisoner volunteers. Things were simpler then. Informed consent was unheard of. No one asked me what I was doing. It was a wonderful time."[15]

The appreciative medical explorer uttering that nostalgic refrain was none other than Albert Montgomery Kligman, the erstwhile *enfant terrible* of the University of Pennsylvania Medical School's Department of Dermatology and one of the busiest prison researchers in postwar America. Considered "brilliant" by many and a "genius" by some, Al Kligman was a whirling dervish of ideas and activity, a man who not only flew planes, rode horses, played tennis, and was able to walk on his hands well into his fifties but was also the author of scores of journal articles on a dizzying array of dermatological subjects and a role model for those who wanted to make money from medicine. An entertaining lecturer and noted raconteur, he had also developed a nationwide reputation for doing human research and was widely envied for having an unlimited supply of test subjects.

The recipient of a Ph.D. in mycology as well as an M.D., Kligman had walked into Holmesburg Prison in 1951 at the request of the institution's medical staff. Beset with another outbreak of athlete's foot, prison personnel thought the Penn professor—a recognized authority on fungus—might be able to provide some helpful suggestions. When he entered the aging prison's large rotunda and saw hundreds of aimless prisoners milling about, Kligman was awestruck. "All I saw before me were acres of skin," he recalled years later of the seminal event. "It was like a farmer seeing a fertile field for the first time."[16]

Kligman immediately recognized what he had—the imprisoned men represented a unique opportunity for unlimited and undisturbed medical research. It was "an anthropoid colony, mainly healthy under perfect control conditions," he told inquiring reporters many years later.

Kligman's farsighted reaction shouldn't be confused with a creative thunderbolt from the heavens; he had been experimenting on retarded children for several years by the time he set foot inside Holmesburg

Prison. Since the mid-1940s Dr. Kligman had been traveling to southern New Jersey to visit the New Jersey State Colonies for the Feebleminded at Vineland and Woodbine to perform various dermatological experiments. In addition to "applying caustic agents" and surgically removing the fingernails of the test subjects, Kligman also "encouraged the development of ringworm by rubbing it in" the "abraded scalp" of the children.[17]

Though some may flinch at such callous treatment of handicapped children, the intrepid young Penn researcher was unmoved. As he told subsequent classes of medical residents of his days at Vineland and Woodbine, "These kids want attention so bad, if you hit them over the head with a hammer they would love you for it."

This cavalier research attitude was brought to Holmesburg in the early 1950s and prevailed there for the next quarter-century. Initially, rudimentary dermatological studies were performed, but even these evolved into something darker and more dangerous for the usually ill-informed test subjects. One 1957 experiment, for example, designed "to promote the inoculation of human skin with . . . ectodermotropic viruses" such as "wart virus . . . herpes simplex and herpes zoster," was reserved for "healthy, colored, male volunteers between the ages of 20 and 45 years of age." Seven of the lucky volunteers received forty-seven inoculations in various parts of their bodies, including the face, scalp, and penis. Another study, just four years later, found "150 white and Negro subjects . . . 21 to 65 years of age" receiving "over 1,000 inoculations" of "cutaneous moniliasis," a skin condition that can cause pain and burning.[18]

Such experiments soon became the order of the day. The endless availability of test subjects—for a dollar a day, no less—and the ability to perform any experiment desired must have been a heady experience. As Kligman once remarked of his good fortune, "I feel almost like a scoundrel—like Machiavelli—because of what I can do to them."

It was during this period that various pharmaceutical companies started to request Phase I trials—large-scale clinical trials of various medicines and other products. Dr. Kligman found the corporate associations, not to mention the remuneration, quite appealing. Fairly soon Holmesburg inmates found themselves involved in a wide array of nontherapeutic experiments testing everything from detergents and deodorants to analgesics and antidepressants.

Eventually Holmesburg would become one of the largest human research factories in America, hosting scores of Phase I studies, mind-control

53

experiments for the U.S. Army, dioxin studies for Dow Chemical, and Kligman's own experiments with radioactive isotopes.[19] In short, Kligman's intellectual curiosity, combined with a knack for entrepreneurial enterprise, transformed an overcrowded city jail into a hotbed of experimental activity. There was something in it for everybody, even the inmates. But it was the inmates who would carry the weight if anything untoward should occur. They alone were saddled with that burden—as Butch Anthony would soon discover.

"He's Got a Body Like Marilyn Monroe"

Butch Anthony's ill-fated decision to become a test subject in Holmesburg Prison's clinical research program would have an immediate and unmistakable impact. It would also profoundly affect his health—both physical and mental—for the rest of his life.

Within minutes of having the "Johnson & Johnson bubble bath" applied to his back and each site covered with gauze pads and adhesive tape, he was unconscious on the cell floor, his cell mates trying to revive him. Soon he was screaming for relief from the intense heat now centered where the foreign substances had been applied.

Over the coming weeks, he was in continuous agony. Minutes seemed like hours and hours like days, as Anthony endured the worst pain and sustained discomfort of his life. The searing, unrelenting heat radiating throughout his back eventually turned his skin red, generated ugly, pus-filled dermal eruptions from head to foot, and made him fear for his very life. Long showers under scalding hot water provided only temporary relief, as the medical personnel on H block—where he had first come in contact with the clinical trials—seemed to have abandoned him. He had been cut loose to fend for himself.

Even his fellow prisoners wanted no part of his situation. Fearing that his appalling condition might be contagious and unnerved by the sight of him, inmates shunned him. Some even threatened him physically if he came too close. Guards eventually ordered him to eat his meals alone in his cell rather than have his disquieting presence trigger a disturbance in the mess hall. Anthony couldn't imagine how he was going to endure much more this.

"I thought I was gonna die," says Anthony. "I really did. There was no relief, and things just seemed to be

5

getting worse. The pain was excruciating, especially under my arms and between my legs. It felt like my whole fuckin' body was reactin'. I felt like something was crawling under my skin. I wasn't sure, but kept thinking it was all due to them spraying my back with that liquid sealer after they put the patches on. I could taste it in my mouth and it immediately made me nauseous, but I really didn't know for sure. The doctors wouldn't see me; they wouldn't talk to me. I couldn't eat in the mess hall anymore. It was fuckin' terrible. All my life I had been quiet, an introvert desiring to stay out of the limelight, and now I was like a neon sign. It just seemed hopeless.

"Even my cell mates wanted to throw me out because I had become such a pain in the ass. They couldn't sleep at night due to all the moaning and screaming I was doin'. Some guys on the block must have thought I was getting fucked or stabbed, I was doin' so much moaning. At night, Youngie and Ruben had to put a white pillowcase or bed sheet on the metal bar we used to open the ceiling vent with and stick it out the cell door to notify the block or center guard that there was a problem in the cell. They wanted me taken to the hospital. They'd tell the guard I was dying and needed to see a doctor. All I ever got was a visit from Otto, another inmate who functioned as the prison nurse. He'd give me a couple of green and yellow pills, something like Emperin, but they didn't really help. Fat Otto got so tired of coming down to my cell at night he started calling me a big baby when he gave me the pills. That would cause me to snap out, start cursing, and lose whatever diplomacy I had left. He didn't know what I was going through. It was unbearable.

"Finally, after about three weeks of this shit, I got some attention. One night about two o'clock in the morning, everybody in the jail is asleep but me, and a guard comes to my cell and opens the door. He calls me out into the corridor and I'm thinking, what now? I get out there and a guy in a business suit is standing out there and he says, 'I'm from the University of Pennsylvania. I heard you're having a problem.'

"I showed him my arms, chest, and face, and said, 'Look what they did to me. Look at this.' I told him I couldn't take much more and said I felt like I was dying.

"He says, 'Come along with me,' and took me over to H block. He takes me into one of the laboratory rooms and tells me to take my clothes off and lay down on the gurney. He then got a gallon bottle of solution and poured it into a basin with a few other things. It had a strong odor and smelled like vinegar. He then got a sponge and started to bathe my body with this vinegar-like solution. He did my entire body from head to foot and then dried me off.

"He then grabbed a set of keys and opened a safe that's on the floor and takes out a small bottle. Now he opens a drawer, takes out a syringe, sticks the needle in the bottle, and draws some of the fluid out. He comes back to me and doesn't say a word. He just shoots that shit in me and almost immediately I felt my whole body relax. It felt like I had been shot up with morphine or heroin. It was strong. He never told me what it was, but I was real mellow after that, and all the pain and itching started to subside. He gave me some cotton balls and some liquid that looked like calamine lotion and told me to apply it three times a day."

Anthony followed the doctor's orders and his condition gradually began to improve. The interminable itching, the alarming redness that had discolored most of his body, and the unrelenting pain slowly diminished in intensity. He could once again eat meals with the other inmates, return to the tailor shop to make prison garments, and finally get something resembling a decent night's sleep. He was on the road to recovery, but not before enduring the worst bout of physical and mental suffering of his life.

All the more perplexing, then, that within weeks of his return to normal he would contemplate another round as an experimental lab rat at Holmesburg Prison.

This most unlikely of scenarios was due to the dangerous and oppressive nature of the environment he found himself in and his susceptibility to suggestion, particularly when counseled by older and presumably wiser associates.

The jail was a hothouse of unbridled emotion, and Anthony was getting his first full dose of it. Up until now he had been in a life-and-death struggle with a malady of unknown origin, one that had preoccupied his every waking moment. Adjusting to the shocking rhythms, dissonant harmonies, and overpowering atmosphere of Holmesburg had been put on hold while he grappled with his catastrophic health problems. Now, however, he was confronted with an equally challenging scenario—the prison culture itself.

"Man, it was like another world. I couldn't believe what went on in there. The noise, the sex, the violence, the pressure, it all just builds until you wanna explode. All day, every day, it was always the same. No letup. No relief. It was terrible. Just the routine alone was difficult to deal with.

"He's Got a Body Like Marilyn Monroe"

"They'd wake us up around six or seven in the morning. You'd hear the guards opening the locks to the cell doors. First you'd hear the electrical switches being thrown and the mashing of the gears that ran above the cell doors for the length of the block. Then you'd hear the guard walking down the block, opening each cell door with that big-ass brass key of his. It looked as big as a man's hand; something like a large factory key on steroids.

"First thing we'd do is pass our trash cans out the door and then go to the shower room on the block and get ourselves a bucket of hot water in order to wash up and brush our teeth. We only had cold water running in our cells so we'd have to wait till morning to get some hot water. Then we'd wait for our blocks to be called down for chow. Usually you'd walk down soup alley with the guys you wanted to sit with in the mess hall, but it didn't always work out that way. There'd be rows of long tables, about three in line and ten or so across, and the guards would make us sit where they wanted us. For breakfast we'd usually get coffee, cereal with powdered milk, or sometimes grits and scrambled eggs, always the powdered variety.

"After about twenty minutes, they'd take us back to our blocks and we'd be called to our different jobs in the jail between 8:00 and 9:00 A.M. I didn't mind having a quick meal, 'cause the chow hall was a place where something could jump off at any moment. You sure as hell didn't wanna be down there among three hundred crazy niggers if something should jump off. I had heard stories about prison riots in the mess hall and what happens when the inmates got ahold of the kitchen and butcher knives. I wanted no parts of it.

"They had a bunch of different jobs in there: a weave shop, a shoe shop, knit shop, tailor shop. Other guys would be working in the laundry or working the officers' mess hall or on cleaning details that were assigned to the visiting room, the receiving room, and things like that.

"I was assigned to the tailor shop. It was upstairs on the second floor, above the scullery. We made prison shirts for the inmates. It was all piece-work. Some guys would be making collars, some guys sleeves, others would be sewing buttons on the shirts and pants. My job was sewing the yokes, or the upper backs of the shirts, onto the rest of the garment. All day long I'd be working this big old sewing machine making shirts for the inmates.

"Around twelve o'clock they'd call us for lunch and we'd have to go back to our block and wait till it was our time to eat. Usually we'd get some watered-down Kool-aid or iced tea and a salami or bologna sandwich. Sometimes we'd get a hot dog. Applesauce was usually the dessert.

"Right after lunch we'd go right back to our job assignments and stay there till around four or five o'clock. It was long hours, and we were only getting twenty-five cents a day, but it kept me off the block. Man, I was thankful for that, 'cause the blocks were a madhouse. I looked for any reason to stay off the block. There was some real crazy shit that went on there.

"Guys would be breaking into other guys' cells and stealing their commissary. Even if they were locked, guys found ways to get into the cells, or guys would just forget to tell the guards to lock their cells when they left the block. And there were some guards who were corrupt and helped inmates steal off of other inmates. It was real corrupt in there.

"They'd usually pick on a guy they figured they could get over on. Someone who was new to the jail and had no friends or homeys to watch his back. Someone who wasn't about to confront anybody about some missing commissary items. These young guys come back to their cells and their whole crib be ripped apart, their commissary taken, and everything of any value gone. They might even see someone wearing something of theirs or eating their commissary, but unless they had a lot of heart they'd just keep their mouths shut. They knew if they confronted someone they'd probably get fucked up. Guys didn't play in there. Everybody had a shank. Or knew where to get one. Holmesburg was a pretty violent place.

59

"I seen guys get beat senseless over nothing. And that sex stuff would really bring out the animal in people. Man, it was like another world. I had heard about them rushin' guys in their cell, but the first time I saw a bunch of them grab a guy, it scared the hell out of me. About five guys rushed a guy in his cell one night, threw a heavy wool blanket over his head, and beat him senseless while they each took turns fucking him. Guys in the corridor knew what was going on but kept their mouths shut. They didn't want the same thing or worse happening to them. The dude didn't have a chance, especially when he can just about breathe with that blanket suffocating him and guys punching him in the head and body. Man, those blanket parties were mean.

"Guys were being beaten bad if they resisted being turned into a homo. Other guys would be talked into it and do what guys wanted them to do. Some young boys who were on their own and had no one watching their back were easy targets for the wolves. Everybody be after them, threatening them, talkin' to 'em, trying to get them to do what they wanted. It was mean, boy. If you couldn't handle yourself or didn't have any homeys around to protect you, you were in trouble.

"He's Got a Body Like Marilyn Monroe"

"I remember the first time I took a shower in the jail. Man, it scared the hell out of me. I'm in the shower room one morning getting washed, and I notice guys were coming in the shower room, but they weren't taking a shower. They'd come in, then go out, and then come back in again. They did the same thing three or four times. Then I heard one of 'em say to the other, 'Hmmm, he's got a body like Marilyn Monroe.' They were talkin' about me. I was the only one in there taking a shower. I got outta there pretty fuckin' quick. They were talkin' about me like I was a naked woman. It freaked me out. I was only twenty or so and didn't have any hair on my face, and these guys were getting off on me. I got paranoid after that and just washed up in my cell. I didn't go back to the shower room for a damn long time after that.

"Some guys were definitely targeted. They'd take a guy and turn him out. And guys would get to accept the life until they went home. Guys would submit. Young boys who were timid and didn't know anybody were in trouble. There'd be guys chasing them and grabbing them like a pack of dogs chasing a rabbit in the park. Then there'd be those guys who thought they were slick, who would cozy up to 'em by speaking soft, talking nice, offering advice, cigarettes, and candy, and then put the moves on them. 'You be my bitch and I'll protect you from the wolves. You turn me down and the brothers will rip the shit out of you.' It was a vicious game, boy. I'm glad I had Youngie and Ruben to watch my back. Without them I don't know what I would have done.

"But there were some old mothers too, guys who had been turned out years ago. Some of them were so female in the way they walked and the way they talked, you would think they were actually women.

"They'd get these guys to actually dress like women. They'd have high-boy collars and wear three-quarter sleeves. They'd even comb their hair like women. Some would even get their hair processed. Guys would be able to come up with a prison version of Congolene that you'd get on the street. They'd get potatoes from the kitchen and lye and soap from the laundry and mash it up real good and mix some other shit in there, and pretty soon Bob, Jim, and Sonny were looking like Valerie, Marvena, and Baby Doll.

"After they would pretty them up, their daddies would solicit them. They'd be pimping them on the blocks. They sold 'em for money, cigarettes, drugs, whatever they wanted or people could afford. A hand job would go for a few cigarettes, a blow job for a pack, and getting fucked would be a carton. They had a whole price list. And there'd be different prices for different hos. Quality was more expensive. The cuter the guy, the more he looked like a girl, the more they could charge.

"Guys would come out of a cell after paying for one of these guys and they'd be bug-eyed and saying, 'Boy, that was mean. Ummm. I gotta get me some more of that.'

"Man, I thought these muthafuckers were crazy. Hell, they'd be moving on guys who didn't even look like a girl.

"I remember this one guy called Flip who looked like a guy but walked and talked like a woman. He was as feminine as any woman and knew how to hide his stuff when he was trying to seduce someone. He'd perfume up his cell and blow talcum powder all over to create this atmosphere. He'd also do some stuff with Wildroot hair cream to kill the smell of feces and make his rectum real smooth and slippery.

"He'd be acting all feminine and telling guys, 'Hey daddy, how you doin'? How's my baby today? Did you like that shot the other day? How'd you like mama to take care of you? Would you like that, baby?'

"Flip did it for cigarettes, candy, whatever. He was known as a top-notch ho. Youngie would send guys over to Flip and tell 'em, 'Mama's got some good pussy.'

"This homosexual thing was nasty. There were a lot of fights and blood bein' shed over homos and who belonged to who in the jail. Guys be yelling, 'That's my homo.' 'Stay the fuck away from her.' 'Keep your fuckin' hands off of her.' Guys would be pimping these guys and some of these crazy muthafuckers would even fall in love with them. Violent fights would jump off over these homos. Lotta guys got stabbed because of this shit.

"You can't believe what went on. And right out in the open. One day I come out of my cell in the morning and I see a line of guys standing in the corridor outside a cell like they're selling lottery tickets or something. There's about ten of 'em standing by the cell door with a blanket over the entrance so you can't see inside. It was one of those mind-your-business things, but it didn't take long to figure out what was going on. They all got cigarettes in their hand and they're ready to pay for service, you know, for sexual favors. They were doin' this boy in there.

"I couldn't believe it. There was a homo in there who was suckin' them off and allowing them to fuck him with his daddy standing at the door collecting the cigarettes like a ticket taker at a movie theater. The dude was younger than me. He may have been about eighteen years old. I never

61

suspected he had those tendencies, but they turned him out. They either beat him up or just the everyday psychological pressure of the joint turned him around.

"This goes on every day before breakfast for almost three weeks. Believe me, those niggers were maniacs. I couldn't believe a little guy could handle all those guys like that. And every day, too. And some of those niggers had horse dicks. I wondered how the fuck some of these niggers could walk around with dicks the size of a Genoa salami. You'd have to strap 'em down with a rope or belt, they were so big. Some of those niggers could have gotten work as Roto-Rooters. I told myself I was cheated by God when I seen what they were packing.

"One day, though, this kid just snaps. He went off. He got so strong he just threw them out of his cell. He even beat up his daddy, who looked like a muscle-bound gorilla. It took a while for the humiliation to come out, but once it did, this kid was a wild man. Once the anger came out of what they had done to him, he just snapped. He took on everybody. They had to come get him and take him off the block.

"But shit like that just happened. It was almost routine. And the guards knew it. Some of them were afraid for themselves. I would see them hide out when things jumped off. I remember a guy going to the guards to complain about some of the shit that was going on and the guard just looked at him and said, 'Look man, I told you to stay up front and not go to the back of the block. Hell, those niggers even tried to fuck me.'

"That sex stuff was deep. It created a whole lot of tension in the jail. I remember one time a guy got so scared from guys peeking at him in his cell, he just snapped. He couldn't take it any longer. He thought they were looking at him like he was a piece of lunchmeat, so he bolted out of there like a scalded dog. He came running down the block screaming his head off. He thought they were gonna come in his cell and fuck him. Guys are coming out to the corridor to see what all the hollerin' is about, and this crazy nigger runs by them in a panic. The whole time he's lookin' over his shoulder to see if they're chasing after him. Well, he ran right into the iron bars that divide the block in half. He knocked himself out cold. He had to be carried out of there on a stretcher. He got paranoid. He couldn't handle the pressure anymore. All he knew was that they were planning on getting him, and he was getting the hell out of there.

"There were some guys on the block you sure as hell didn't want to mess with. G block had some of the toughest guys in the jail. All the big dudes who worked in the boiler room and those in the coal gang was on my block. These guys ate bricks. They were tough, muscle-bound killers. I said, 'How the hell did I get put on this block? I don't belong here.'

"Even the little guys, though, could handle themselves and do a lot of damage. Some of those guys being pressured for sex turned out to be nasty muthafuckers. They wouldn't take that bullshit. They wouldn't be turned out. They fought back. I saw a little guy fightin' one of these big dudes over some of this sex stuff. He was doing okay until the big guy finally got the upper hand and started to do a number on him. The little guy got away and ran back to his cell. But he came flying back with a razor blade between his fingers. He went after the big guy swinging his hand like a machete. He sliced that big muthafucker pretty bad. He was bleeding like a monster. Must have cut him about ten times, mostly in the face and head. Guards came running and whistles and sirens start going off. It was wild. They finally pulled the guys apart, but there was blood all over the place. I'm tellin' you, the Burg was bad. The tension was tremendous.

"Some of this stuff was even happening on H block, where they did the experiments. Guys were being hustled over there. It was a big scam. It made it that much worse 'cause the doctors and the university were supposed to be over there doing important stuff. Guys who put out were getting on the better tests and making all that money. I even heard some of 'em were getting paid and weren't even on the tests. That's how corrupt it had become. It was money for sex.

"And they were selling a lot of swag as well. I remember inmate workers for the U of P were getting ahold of some of the old baby food bottles that were tested on the inmates and filling 'em with two-hundred-proof whole grain alcohol. Then they'd sell the bottles to the inmates for a carton of cigarettes. Guys would then pay kitchen workers for a quart can of orange juice and go out in the yard and party. They'd be making screwdrivers out in the yard. Some of 'em came back in the jail drunk as hell. They were fucked up. But that's what went on in there. Holmesburg was a madhouse."

Edward Anthony's recollections of Holmesburg Prison are not the product of a highly imaginative mind suffering periodic flights of fancy. The city's oldest jail was notorious for both brutality and cunning scams. Even the correctional officers paid to work there hated it and were constantly putting in requests for a transfer. A double shift anywhere else was better than doing eight hours at the Burg. The House of Correction and the

Detention Center, located nearby, had many of the same types of criminals confined in them, but the burglars, rapists, and murderers incarcerated in Holmesburg always seemed worse: more threatening, more menacing, more difficult to manage. There was something different about Holmesburg. Everyone and everything was always in your face. It was just more intense—the cold in the winter seemed colder, the heat in the summer felt more searing, the interpersonal relationships, more explosive. The simmering anger and resentment that pervaded Holmesburg seemed to envelop the cell blocks and everyone who inhabited them.

Anthony's descriptions of violence and forbidden sex on the blocks are not the imaginings of a windy Hollywood publicity agent hawking a sleazy porno film. Those incidents and more really occurred there.[1] Though the Burg's hostile and sexually predatory atmosphere was known firsthand only to those unfortunate enough to pass through the institution, the general public got its first whiff of the villainous mayhem going on behind those ominous stone walls in the summer of 1968, when two slightly built inmates, nineteen and twenty-one years old, admitted in court that they had been repeatedly raped inside the county jail. Stunned by the allegations—and no doubt further spurred by the media's alarmed reaction—Judge Alexander F. Barbieri appointed District Attorney Arlen Specter's top assistant, Alan Davis, to investigate the troubling allegations.[2]

Davis and his staff initiated a vigorous investigation into the city's penal system, giving particularly close scrutiny to Holmesburg's prior two years of operation. More than thirty-three hundred of the sixty thousand inmates who passed through the three-prison system during that time were interviewed, as were 561 custody personnel. After an intense investigation that included scores of polygraph examinations, investigators found that "sexual assaults in the Philadelphia Prison System" were of "epidemic" proportions. According to the report,

> Virtually every slightly built young man committed by the courts is sexually approached within a day or two after his admission to prison. Many of these young men are repeatedly raped by gangs of inmates. Others, because of the threat of gang rape, seek protection by entering into a homosexual relationship with an individual tormentor. Only the tougher and more hardened young men and those few so obviously frail that they are immediately locked up for their own protection, escape homosexual rape.[3]

The report went on to describe how victims were selected, methods of attack, and how such disturbing acts of violence could go undetected by the authorities. After many months of examining all the evidence, investigators calculated the "true number of assaults . . . was actually about 2,000."

Though it came as no surprise to inmates like Eddie Anthony, the report shocked many readers by focusing attention on the deleterious impact of the University of Pennsylvania's medical research program. Underscoring the point that "a person with economic advantage in prison often uses it to gain sexual advantage," the Davis report argued that the "large laboratory on H block" managed by the University of Pennsylvania had a terrible effect on the daily operations of the prison. "Disproportionate wealth in the hands of a few inmates," the report said, "leads to favoritism, bribery, and jealousy among the guards, resulting in disrespect for supervisory authority and prison regulations." Furthermore, the medical research program "contributed to homosexuality in the prison."

The report also profiled the nefarious maneuverings of an imprisoned con man who had ingratiated himself with the Penn researchers and thereby attained "power to decide which inmates would serve as subjects on various tests." With his "special taste for newly admitted young males," this inmate medical technician was able to pick any of them as "cell mates for as long as he wished" and then "solicited them to engage in sexual acts in return for him giving them a steady stream of luxuries and for getting them on the tests." This one sex-for-money scheme was estimated to have paid out $10,000 to $20,000 a year—money supplied by the University of Pennsylvania and its various contractors.

The Davis report and the subsequent salacious newspaper headlines— "Lab Testing Program Tied to Prison Sex Corruption," for example—caught the attention of city officials, but it would be years before the mayor and the prison system's board of trustees seriously confronted the complex web of issues presented by the human research program it was hosting.

The many men and women incarcerated in the Philadelphia Prison System who chose to become part of the medical research program were no better than throwaway people, part of the conveyor belt of research subjects used for exploitation and experimentation. Desperate, ill informed, and easily taken advantage of, they had little recourse if something went wrong.

Though he was well aware of the dangers, Edward Anthony was once again contemplating subjecting himself to science.

"They Called Me Outer Limits"

"I was doing better physically, but I was broke. My skin had practically returned to normal, and I started thinking about another test. I had only got $37 for that first test, and it was now long gone. I was making twenty-five cents a day in the tailor shop, and that was working from eight in the morning till four in the afternoon. It added up to nothing. My family did as they said and sent me a money order once in a while, but it was only for $6. It wasn't very much, but at least they were now communicating with me.

"In the meantime, everybody else in the jail is making money on the tests. They had every kind of test you could think of. The jail was really about testing. You know, getting paid. Both Ruben and Youngie were encouraging me to get on a test. They were on tests and not getting hurt. They were making money and not having any problems. They were selective, though, in what they got involved with. They were doing diet tests, dandruff shampoos, even a margarine test. Youngie was being given so much margarine to eat, he started to grease his skin with it. He used it as a skin moisturizer. Everybody in the jail was on them and making money. You had to if you wanted to survive. Do you know what it's like when everybody seems to have stuff and you don't? You know what it's like when folks are throwing a party and you ain't invited? I just wanted to get into the flow of things and started to try and find another test where I wouldn't get fucked up.

"I know I said that's it, fuck it, I'd never take another test after I recovered from that first one, but jail does things to you. You really needed money to be independent in there. You're vulnerable in there with all that crazy shit going on, the fights, the sex, the robbing that was going on. Those tests allowed you to make some money. You try to build up a shield and don't want to be sucked into bad stuff because you need something. The only ones not on the tests were those guys with money and the followers of Elijah Muhammad. The Black Muslims said whitey was the devil and the white man would fuck you up. They wanted no parts of whitey or his doctors. Just about anybody outside of them, though, was on the tests. You knew you were rolling the dice with your health, but guys were willing to take the chance. We were desperate.

"Youngie was on a milkshake test at the time and periodically going down to H block, and he comes back all excited one day and says, 'Hey Butch, they got a study paying $30 for just three days. They shoot some dye in you and monitor your reaction for three days in a trailer they got at the end of the block, and then you're done. You'll get better food, and they even got a television in the trailer you can watch.'

"The next day I went down to H block and said, 'I heard you're lookin' for guys for the dye study.'

"The day after I signed up, they called me down. There were five of us, and they told us to bring our belongings. Things like cigarettes, candy, deodorant, a washcloth, and toothpaste. They took us to the end of the block, where they had a small trailer that contained bunk beds. Each of us was assigned a bed and we were told to take off our clothes and put on one of those little hospital smocks that are open in the back. They then shot a clear liquid in us. They did it intravenously in a vein. You could taste it immediately. It tasted oily, almost like butter, and your body felt warm, like it was melting. Each day we got one of these intravenous shots. Then they'd take blood from us and keep us hooked up to some electronic monitors. We were never told what the purpose of all this was, just that it was some kind of dye test.

"It was okay. I never had any negative reaction to this test. Compared to that first test, it was just like drinking water. After the third day they just said we could go back to our own block, and after a few more days we got a receipt for $30. I now had money on the books. It felt better having some money like the rest of the inmates. I went to commissary and bought a big box of potato chips, Hershey bars with almonds, ice cream, cigarettes, and movie tickets. I could live again. I could lay back now and not worry about borrowing from somebody and one of these asshole bandits coming on to me. In fact, I could loan guys stuff and then get repaid when I was short. Now I could be like the others and enjoy myself, or as much as one could in jail.

"I waited a good two months before I did another test. My money was running low, and guys were encouraging me to do another one. I know I should have been more cautious after what happened to me the first time, but I was young and wild. I was a functional illiterate who didn't know any better. Besides, I didn't have any trouble with the dye test. And it felt damn good to have some money. I wasn't like some guys who didn't have a cent, or those who were being helped out by asshole bandits who were looking to get repaid with certain favors. I knew I wasn't gonna go that way if I could help it.

"One day Youngie comes back from H block all excited and starts telling me about a government test that's paying big money. There were several parts to the test, and the first part alone was paying $50. He said everybody was talking about it and that I should get on it.

"It sounded pretty good to me, too. I thought the government would take care of us. I trusted them; you know, G. I. Joe and all that. My older brothers had been in the service and it had been okay, except Wilbert had come back from Korea a drug addict. When they came down the block that night giving out medication and looking for volunteers, I put my name on the list, but the inmate recruiter said the money was so good they had more guys than they needed and they might not need me.

"The next day, though, I was one of the guys that got called down. There was a large group of us, about fifteen to twenty guys. They sat us down around a table and explained that we were gonna do the first part of the test, and those that did well would go on to the second part. The first part was really nothing at all; it just consisted of doing math problems in a certain amount of time. There were a whole lot of simple addition, subtraction, and multiplication problems on the sheet of paper they gave us. Guys really got excited when they heard that for each problem we got right they'd give us ten cents. The ten cents really sounded good, since we were only making a quarter a day in most of our jobs. There were approximately a hundred problems on the sheet, and I guess they gave us around fifteen minutes to do them. When time was up, they collected all the papers.

"They said we were now gonna take another math test, but before we did they wanted us to drink something. They gave all of us a two-ounce paper cup filled with a clear liquid, and we drank it. After waiting a while, I guess for the solution to take effect, they handed out another piece of paper filled with math problems.

"They said 'go' and started to time us, but to tell you the truth, I don't know if I even did two or three of the problems. Things started to move, everything seemed magnified, and the room seemed to be moving like water. Noise from the prison loudspeaker made me think of a foghorn on a ship at sea. I couldn't concentrate. Things were getting blurry. The walls were moving. I was trippin'.

"Some of the guys were doing problems like it was nothing and may have finished the test, but I wasn't one of them. I was looking around, and a couple other guys were just like me, spaced out. I don't even remember how I got back to my block. I was trippin', man. They never called me back after that. I guess they were testing to see how sensitive you were to the stuff before they put you in the trailer where the really heavy stuff was being given out.

"After drinking that stuff, I got paranoid. I was fucked up. I didn't trust anybody. I didn't trust myself. I thought guys were whispering about me, looking at me, conspiring to do something to me. I stopped smoking cigarettes from packages and started smoking butts I picked up off the cell floor. I used to be talkative and play chess with guys, but now I became reclusive and went into a shell. I wouldn't talk to anybody. My cell mates were scared of me. I'd lie in my cell, never say anything, and then all of a sudden I'd break out laughing. Or people be laughing at a joke and I'd break out laughing ten minutes later. My cell mates wanted me taken out of the cell. They wanted me put in OBS [observation unit for the mentally disturbed]. It got so bad, guys on the block started calling me 'Outer Limits.'

"I wouldn't let anybody get close to me, even Youngie and Ruben, who I knew from the neighborhood and had been watching my back in there. That shit had me going. Those muthafuckin' doctors had done it to me again. I was hearing voices, seeing things, and just stayed in my cell on the block for days, maybe weeks. I don't know how much time went by. I just laid there and hallucinated. I thought I was in hell. I didn't want to see a doctor or anybody. I was in my own little world.

"This shit they gave me turned my whole life around. I was normally friendly and outgoing, and all of a sudden I was fearful and angry all the time. I'd hear guys talkin' and think they were talkin' about me. I always thought they were going to do something to me. I'd ball my hands up into a fist and start muttering like I was gonna beat the hell out of someone. I actually punched one guy in the face who had been a friend of mine, just because I thought he was going to do something to me. But he wasn't. I hit him for nothing. I couldn't distinguish nothing from nothing. Guys would look at me and then at each other and say, 'This muthafucker is crazy.' Ruben and Youngie wanted me gone. There were other guys like me who were taken to OBS and put on break fluid [Thorazine]. Guys on those tests were coming out of the army trailers like zombies. I wasn't much better. I was a mess. Everybody knew I had snapped. They all started calling me 'Outer Limits.' They'd come up to Youngie or Ruben and ask, 'How's Outer Limits today? He any better?'

The residents of G block obviously saw a similarity between one of their own and the strange characters appearing on the popular science fiction television show that captivated viewers with an array of extraterrestrial aliens and bizarre, futuristic story lines. The year was 1964, and Butch Anthony would certainly not be the only Holmesburg inmate to have his personality altered by the U.S. Army's psychochemical trials. It is more than likely that Anthony was one of the earliest subjects of what would eventually become known—to black inmates at least—as the controversial "pay me no mind list" experiments.

The odd, unscientific designation was given to those mind-altering clinical trials that resulted in many prisoners who left the army trailers— which had been specifically placed inside prison walls for these sensitive psychotropic drug studies—not knowing their own names, where they were, or what had happened to them. Totally divorced from reality in some instances and unable to care for themselves, they were forced to wear badges on their prison jumpsuits identifying them as University of Pennsylvania/U.S. Army experimental volunteers, to be handled with care. Apparently it wasn't all that unusual to see inmates staring into space, mumbling incoherently, or just walking around the jail like zombies.

Holmesburg Prison at the time was a seventy-year-old, underfunded, overcrowded city jail that had become a key building block in America's chemical warfare arsenal. For the next decade, the prison would play a critical role not only in the military's hunt for incapacitating chemical substances, but also in the CIA's longtime search for a designer drug that could create a "Manchurian candidate."[1]

The county lockup in Philadelphia first appeared on the army's radar screen in the early 1960s, when its investigation of incapacitating chemical agents shifted from LSD to an assortment of belladonna-like compounds that could "produce temporary military ineffectiveness without permanent injury or death." The task was a difficult one, as few pharmacological substances seemed capable of performing this role. Unlike LSD, chemicals like atropine, scopolamine, belladonna, and various benzilates "revealed in humans a considerable variation in the time of onset and duration." Scopolamine, for example, "produced effects within minutes, but lasted only a few hours, while a benzilate produced peak central nervous system effects at about eight hours and had a delirious effect for 24 to 72 hours."[2]

Because of the "unusually long effects" of certain substances, it was determined that the compound deserved greater study. There was one problem, however. Edgewood Arsenal in Maryland, the home of the U.S. Army's Chemical Corps, was a relatively small base and lacked the additional testing capacity required for this new round of studies. Moreover, because of the potency of the chemical agents under review, a test subject needed to remain under observation longer than a soldier's two-month assignment to Edgewood would allow. Anxious to find a university-centered research facility along the eastern seaboard, the army engaged the University of Pennsylvania, which already had a widely recognized reputation in the field of human research. Dr. Albert Kligman and Holmesburg Prison were well-established names in the world of human research and clinical trials.[3]

As far back as the early 1950s, Penn and the army had entered into a series of contractual relationships to evaluate the impact of certain drugs on humans. The first, in 1951, "The Study of Chemical Warfare Casualties in Man," was a laboratory study. Subsequent experimental studies used volunteers, but their origin is difficult to determine.[4] By 1964, however, government documents disclose prison inmates as the test subjects and Holmesburg as the test site.

"Threshold Doses in Humans and Evaluation of Drugs in Man" incorporated hundreds of Holmesburg inmates as experimental volunteers. Designed to test a dizzying assortment of chemicals, including ditran, atropine, scopolamine, and other glycolate agents, the study, the army hoped, would refine its knowledge of incapacitants that affected the central nervous system. Depending on the dosage, test subjects could practically count on "delirium, physical in-coordination, blurred vision, inhibition of sweating and salivation, rapid heart rate, elevated blood pressure, increased body temperature, and at high doses, vomiting, prostration, and stupor or coma."[5]

Documents disclose that, depending upon the particular study, test subjects were given a battery of tests, including the Wechsler Adult Intelligence Scale, Bender-Gestalt, and the Thematic Apperception Test, as well as a number facility test designed to monitor cognitive performance. The army concluded that paying inmates a few cents for each correct answer, and a little more after receiving an investigational drug, instilled "a high level of motivation in this population." As one Holmesburg research assistant said, "We never tried to appeal to their sense of patriotism or altruism. We told them this was a test you could make some money on."[6]

Inmate reaction to the studies varied widely. Some prisoners were unfazed by the drugs, which were usually administered orally or by injection or aerosol mist, while others behaved in potentially violent ways. For example, while one chemically injected inmate snoozed through his test, another became enraged, tore a bolted toilet fixture from the floor, and proceeded to crash through the cell door. As the army psychopharmacologist in charge of the experiment recalled years later, "I was pretty sure he would be menacing. He was a monster of a man, 250 pounds of muscle. He blew the door right off the hinges, and they were pretty solid, well-built trailers. I was standing there pretty stunned."[7]

Such episodes, along with the far more common hallucinogenic reactions, where test subjects envisioned "giant ants and spiders coming out of the walls," and their subsequent stuporous aftermath, gave the army experiments an infamous reputation in the jail. Inmates wanted the money the better-paying army experiments provided, but the terrifying visions and lengthy recovery period scared many of them off.

For those who thought they were invulnerable or found the temptation of the money irresistible, the army trials could prove a stressful psychological ordeal. Edward "Butch" Anthony was now going through just such an ordeal.

"I'm tellin' you, I wanted to die. This test had me so fucked up I just wanted to die. In that first experiment, the patch test that affected my skin and hurt so bad, I was afraid I was gonna die. But this one did such strange stuff to my head, I really *wanted* to die. I was thinkin' about killing myself. I'm serious; it was so bad I had visions of me killing myself.

"I couldn't handle it anymore. I didn't want to see any doctors. Didn't want to see anybody. I thought guys were plotting to get me, guys out to hurt me. I was paranoid. I wasn't the same person anymore.

"A good example of that was when my wife came up to the prison for a visit. I don't know for sure what I looked like or how I acted, but it must have been bad. I walked into the visiting area, and not too much time went by before she started crying and sobbing, 'What's wrong with you?'

'What's happened to you?' 'What did they do to you?' She left the prison crying way before our time was up. I tried to talk to her, but I must have looked and sounded pretty bad. She leaned toward the screen that separated us to get a better look at me and just walked out. She left with tears streaming down her face.

"That started everything off. It got bad pretty quick after that. Next thing I know, I'm being called out for another visit. It must have been only a day or two later. I rarely got visits, so this was really unusual. It was my mother, who had come up on a special visit to see me, to check me out after talking to my wife. I go down there and she starts screaming, 'Look at you. What are you doing in there? You're doing drugs again, aren't you? I want you to get out of that cell with Youngie and them. Why are you doin' drugs in here? That is what got you in here in the first place. Those damn drugs, I want you to get away from Youngie and put in another cell. Look at you, you look a mess.'

"She made such a commotion in the visiting area, they took me away and put me back on the block. She figured Youngie was giving me drugs. In her eyes he was an older guy and a bad seed in the neighborhood. He must be influencing me. She must have been hot, 'cause she went to see the warden. It wasn't long after that that I'm getting called to report to center. They tell me to go to Major Turley's office, so I know something bad is going down. His office is right off of center, and he comes down on me right away when I go in there.

"'Who's bringing the drugs in to you?'

"'Nobody,' I say. 'I ain't doing drugs.'

"Turley says, 'I asked you, who are you getting the drugs from?'

"'No one,' I tell him.

"'Don't lie to me, Anthony,' he says.

"He then brings over a whole set of pictures, photographs of all the kitchen workers who are housed on A block, and starts asking me, 'Which one was it? Who gave you the drugs?'

"'None of them did,' I tell him. 'The only drugs I got were from the University of Pennsylvania.'

"'If you don't cooperate,' Turley says, 'it's going to be bad for you. We'll send you to the penitentiary.'

"I sure don't wanna be a snitch, especially when none of the guys he's showing me photographs of did anything wrong. But he didn't believe me. They thought somebody was slipping me some prison swag that I was getting fucked up on. They couldn't understand it was their own damn prison experiments that were messing people up.

"They write me up and send me to one of their disciplinary hearings. The inmates called it kangaroo court 'cause you didn't have a chance. In the hearing room are Major Turley, Lieutenant Fromhold, and a couple of guards. There's no one representing me there but me. It only took a couple of minutes for them to find me guilty.

"They threw me in the hole for ten days. Man, I thought I was in hell. They put me in one of their worst punishment cells, ones with no lights, no toilet, no windows or anything; just blackness all the time. They stripped me naked except for a pair of underpants, a coarse wool blanket they threw at me, a thin plastic mattress that was on the floor, and a metal bucket to piss and shit in.

"It was bad. I did push-ups all day long. I was paranoid and didn't want to hear my own brain. I couldn't sleep, and my mind would think of all kinds of crazy shit. I blamed myself for getting in such a mess. I should have learned the first time not to trust the doctors. Doctors were dangerous. And I was a glutton for punishment. I punished myself on the street and now I was doing it in prison, too, by getting on those tests. I was rolling the dice on those doctors being humane human beings, but they weren't. They were vampires. They just hurt me.

"I started to reflect on what was going on and all the pain I had to endure because of these tests. It took so long for them to pay attention to me, to see that I needed help. It was as if they threw me under the rug and forgot about me. The doctors didn't care. The guards didn't care. It was supposed to be a humane society, but it wasn't. I thought I had done something very wrong in my life to deserve the treatment I was getting.

"I started to doubt there was a God. How could he let these things happen to me? I thought I was going crazy. I couldn't stop thinking about it. I just did the push-ups to distract myself from thinking.

"The only contact I had with other humans was when they brought my food. I got a cup of coffee in the morning with two pieces of bread, and in the afternoons they gave me a cup of iced tea and two more pieces of bread. At night I got a half a meal. Man, I just wanted to die. No light, no windows, things crawling around on the floor. I could hear and feel them, but it was so dark I couldn't see them. It was terrible. And all this for something I didn't even do. They were the ones who did it to me.

"After the ten days were up, they took me out of the hole and put me back in my cell with Ruben and Youngie. I came back to a pretty warm reception. Guys on the block were glad to see me and expressed their concern, but I was still standoffish. Not as bad as I had been before, but still uncomfortable. I kept to myself and just stayed away from people.

"It really wasn't until a little while later that I snapped out of it. I was lying on the bed in my cell one day and heard somebody playing congas on the block. I loved playing the congas as a kid and played with some decent groups as a teenager. I went over to the guy's cell where the music was coming from and he let me play with him for a while. Playing the congas brought me back as Butch. I started to be myself again, friendly, talkative, and outgoing, or as much as you can be in prison. I had finally come back to what I was really like. I was no longer the guy they called Outer Limits."

"Fruit Up"

As he gradually returned to normal in the aftermath of the army's chemically induced personality transformation, Butch wasn't exactly returning to the most supportive or soothing of recuperative environments. He was still on a raucous cell block in a dangerous big-city jail that presented a psychological challenge to the most sane and seasoned of criminal warriors. If the loss of one's freedom, bad food, hostile guards, rival gangs, and the ever-present threat of rape weren't enough to make one fearful of losing one's sanity, the jail was always capable of coming up with a few more horrors. Holmesburg, in fact, had cornered the market on clinical trials. The place—especially for the unanointed—was an experimental showcase of strange sights and medical oddities that was made all the more dramatic by its setting in a dilapidated and malodorous fortress.

Though Butch was now a veteran of the human research studies, the experience of seeing one's fellow man—or, in Holmesburg's case, hundreds of men—in unusual and sometimes dire physical circumstances was still unnerving. Just being a spectator could boggle the mind.

"Even walking through center and going by H block could be upsetting," recalls Butch. "Guys would be strapped and wrapped with all sorts of things. I seen guys wearing metal cups on their foreheads and other guys who had little cups taped inside their legs next to their testicles. Then there were guys who had their feet wrapped in plastic and were told to wear heavy army boots twenty-four hours a day. Guys would be sitting around with their hands and arms in large cans of liquid. They were told they were involved in testing new soap powders and detergents, but some of those guys came out with some pretty damaged skin. That wasn't any kind of detergent I ever seen.

"There were all kinds of strange things going on over there. It scared the hell out of me. I remember being over there one morning and I saw a ladder with a toilet seat on top of it. And behind the toilet seat was a camera. I said to one of the inmate medical technicians, 'What kind of test is this?' and he said it was set up to 'take pictures of someone defecating.' Another time I was over there and I seen a guy take his shirt off, and he was growing breasts like a woman. I said, 'What kind of test is this?' and he said it was a 'hormone test.' They were giving guys hormones that were turning their whole nature around. Man, it was deep."

If that wasn't bad enough, some of the results of the U.S. Army's chemical warfare studies were even more bizarre.

"Some dudes went clear out of their mind," says Anthony. "My experience was mild compared to some of the guys who came out of those army trailers. Some guys would be out in the yard standing and walking around like zombies. They'd just stare into space. The guards would have to go out and get them and bring them back inside. Other guys would go to the wrong block and get in fights, or hold up the line in the mess hall 'cause they could no longer make up their mind. Their power to make decisions was gone.

"Lotta guys would get paranoid and ball their hands into a fist and look like they were gonna punch somebody. And some did and would have to be dragged off by the goon squad and put in cells with four-point restraints. Some of those guys wouldn't know their own strength and would tear the metal and leather bindings loose. The guards would then have to call the doctors to come and shoot them up with Thorazine or Haldol to shut them down. Once they were hit with brake fluid, they were really out of it. I'm telling you, a lot of guys who went through those army experiments ended up in OBS because of the hallucinating and paranoia. Yeah, Holmesburg became a house of horrors."

Butch's way of dealing with the wide range of bizarre and menacing stimuli surrounding him was to stay close to home—he rarely left his cell. His prison job, mess hall, and occasional few minutes in a fellow inmate's cell to play the congas were the only times he'd vacate his cell. The cautious routine, however, brought him an unexpected bonus—Butch finally learned how to read.

"All my life I was a functional illiterate," says Anthony matter-of-factly. "I got to eleventh grade but could only read the tiniest of words and couldn't hardly write anything at all. My sisters used to say to me, 'Butch, how can you be so dumb?' when they were helping me with my schoolwork. I was slow at everything when it came to reading and writing. But in school they kept on promoting me to the next grade.

"It always troubled me that I couldn't read like other people, but it really got to bothering me when I was locked up in a cell with Youngie and Ruben. I'd see them reading books at night and talking about what they were reading, and I couldn't participate. I'd just listen to them and wish I could have done the same thing. I really felt inferior that I couldn't do what everyone else was able to do.

"They even had to help me write letters to my wife. Laura was always writing letters to me. They were really nice, sweet letters telling me how she missed me and hoping I was getting along all right. I could read most of 'em, and Youngie and Ruben would help me with the words I didn't know, but I couldn't reply. I never wrote her back. I couldn't. I didn't know enough words. It would've sounded really immature if I would have written letters to her.

"I finally asked Youngie to help me. He was smart and could really whip that shit out. He was a great talker and could write really good letters. I'm sure Laura knew it wasn't me writing those letters to her, but at least she knew I was thinking of her.

"Then one day Youngie got off work early and came back to the block and caught me in the cell looking at one of his books, *She,* by A. J. Rodgers. The guys were always talking about things that were happening in this book and I wanted to appreciate it too.

"'What the hell you doing with that book, nigger?' said Youngie between laughs. 'You know you can't read.'

"'Yeah,' I replied, 'but I can try.'

"He saw I was having trouble with the big words, so he pulled out one of his books and threw it to me. It was a dictionary. It had been in the cell all that time, but it didn't mean nothin' to me. I had never used one before, so he showed me how to use it to look up words, their meanings, and how they are spelled. That book opened a whole new world to me. I started reading all the time and began going to ABE [Adult Basic Education] classes for reading, writing, and arithmetic.

"I started reading novels like the other guys on the block and was now able to take part in discussions guys would have about what they were reading. I read anything I could get my hands on and was always in the prison library looking for stuff. With the help of the dictionary I was able to

79

read anything I wanted. I could read pages from a book and it would be like scenes from a movie. I could now picture things I was reading just as if I was in a movie theater.

"I even started writing letters. I felt more confident with all the new words I was learning and books I was reading. I started writing letters to Laura and she loved them. She had never received real letters from me, ones I had wrote myself. I was writing her two, three times a week. This was after I had Youngie send her two he had written for me months earlier. Now she was getting them directly from me. It was beautiful.

"I got so good at it, other guys on the block who couldn't write their own letters to their wives or girlfriends would come to me. They'd say, 'Butch, you're good at writin' letters. I'll give you a pack or two of cigarettes if you'll write me a joint to my old lady.' In no time at all it seemed I was writing letters for half the guys on the block. I was making two, three, sometimes four packs per letter, and I never got a complaint. I became a Casanova in the mail.

"In fact, I got so good, other guys' wives started to fall in love with me. One guy said his wife came up to the jail for a visit and demanded to know who wrote the letter. She told her husband, 'I want to see the nigger who wrote this. I want to see him. Bring him here.' Yeah, I became a real mailbox Valentino. I really became inspired, because I didn't know I had such a gift."

At about the same time, Butch found another outlet for his nascent educational and artistic interests—music. The therapeutic role played by the congas in his recovery from the army experiments also rekindled his interest in music, particularly jazz. He had long been a devotee of Miles Davis, John Coltrane, and Dave Brubeck, and he eventually discovered that Holmesburg had a small but spirited collection of musicians who hung out at the band room on A block. Butch managed to get a pass from Vern, a friend from the Village who ran the band room, and found a home alongside some musically gifted, like-minded inmates. Appreciative but unschooled in the rudiments of making music with anything outside the percussion family, he decided to try his hand with a wind instrument, a trombone.

Butch practiced for hours each day, obediently took direction from his more musically gifted mentors, and was inspired by his talented new associates. Just being around creative men who were directed toward something other than getting high or in trouble on the block was a refreshing change.

The band room became for Butch an oasis of expressive freedom and spiritual rejuvenation in a gloomy, steel-and-cinderblock wasteland.

"We had some dynamite musicians," says Anthony of his bandmates. "There were guys in there who had played with Monk, guys who played the sax like Bird and Getz and the trumpet like Miles. Jake Garrett was a great bass player and had played with Dakota Staton, and Jerome Stennett had played with Jimmy Heath. Ernie Dunkin could play the hell out of the sax and had once played with Horace Silver. Those guys could really play, and it was inspiring just being around them. They gave shows in the gym during holidays like Thanksgiving and Christmas, and the guys in the jail really loved it. They were hearing some really fine musicians play. I was never good enough to perform with them, but just being around those guys and practicing with them was enjoyable. Even though I was in jail and missed my wife, I was learning something I never did on the street. Reading, writing, and learning to play music opened up a whole new world for me. I'm not saying there weren't times when I wouldn't have minded a cozy bed, a shot of heroin, and a couple dozen Charlie Parker records, but more and more I started seeing I had more potential than being a junkie and street hustler, which is what I was. I was beginning to realize I could actually make something out of myself."

It should be no surprise if Butch Anthony's latent appreciation of a good dictionary and the arts behind prison bars resembled that of another, more famous high school dropout with a history of narcotics and criminal activity. Many prisoners, in fact, had followed the path of self-realization and self-improvement personified by Malcolm X during his time in Norfolk Prison in Massachusetts more than a decade earlier.[1] "Barely literate and addicted to various drugs," Malcolm Little had become alienated from his Baptist roots and was serving a seventy-seven-month sentence for burglary and larceny when he came into contact with the teachings of Elijah Muhammad and the Nation of Islam.[2] Muhammad's "kindness and understanding," moral guidance, and philosophical framework for understanding the white man's historic oppression of blacks attracted not only Malcolm but thousands of other African American men sitting on barren cell blocks across America.

Though partially based on smatterings of Moorish science, Father Divine's peace mission, and orthodox Islam, along with a bizarre combination of additional concepts and mythical creations (including alien life, evil

81

scientists, exploding planets, and a heavily armed "technological monstrosity called the Mother Plane"), the Nation of Islam's unique take on cosmology, and its promotion of black self-help and black separatism, had strong appeal for certain segments of a persecuted and long-suffering people.[3]

Despite the success Fard Muhammad and Elijah Muhammad had recruiting NOI adherents on the street, they discovered even better recruitment venues. Prisons, for instance, became particularly successful sites for their human fishing expeditions from the 1950s to the 1970s—especially when the NOI minister or recruiter was as dynamic a personality as Malcolm X. Although the prohibition against drinking, smoking, and fornication may have deterred some potential converts, black prisoners in striped prison garb, ankle chains, and little to look forward to often found it easy to adopt a "racially chauvinistic" religion that excoriated "white devils" for all the black man's problems.

Organized in strict paramilitary fashion, with imams (religious leaders), captains, and soldiers ("Fruit of Islam"), the Nation of Islam could often appear a cohesive and autonomous governmental unit—even though they were inmates confined behind thirty-five-foot walls. In some urban jails, members of the Nation wouldn't take orders from a correctional officer until an FOI official had sanctioned it. Just witnessing a couple dozen FOI members marching in military fashion from a cell block to a gym or mess hall could give one a chill, not to mention watching what happened to an "infidel" (an enemy of the Nation) targeted for retribution by the messenger's army.[4]

Philadelphia's prison system was a particularly violent hotbed of Muslim recruitment and aggression. Although Elijah Muhammad, in his public pronouncements, called for abstemious behavior and moral rectitude from his followers, the members of Temple No. 12 in North Philadelphia would eventually become known for their drug activity and killing sprees.[5] Nearly all of the founding ringleaders of the Black Mafia, as the gang would eventually be known, were members in good standing at Temple No. 12. They were also graduates of Holmesburg. When crimes were committed and police were in hot pursuit, it was not unusual to learn that the wanted individuals were being safely quartered in Muslim mosques around the country. When the suspects were eventually captured and brought to trial, prosecutors had trouble winning convictions because key witnesses were often murdered before they could testify.

If people on Philadelphia's streets felt threatened by criminal elements in the Nation of Islam, one can only imagine the pressure inmates felt inside the walls of Holmesburg Prison. Pressure to join the Fruit of Islam only compounded the many pressures with which inmates already contended, making for a truly frightening scenario. Many abandoned their religious reservations, swore a declaration of faith, and became jailhouse Muslims. Others rejected the invitation to join, but sometimes paid the price.

"I was by myself, practicing the trombone," says Butch, "when they first approached me. Youngie and Ruben had told me to stay clear of the Muslims, but I was alone in the cell when they came calling, and they were pretty respectful. 'Brother,' said one of the men, 'you care to come to a meeting tonight?'

"'What kind of meeting?' I asked. 'What's it about?'

"'It's about you,' he said. 'It's about you living in a wilderness of lies and deceit. Come tonight and learn how to find your way out of this hell you're in.'

"I didn't really know what he was talking about, but I didn't want to offend them. I knew a little about their rep in the jail and knew you could have a serious problem if you crossed the brothers. I had heard about incidents when a Muslim imam or captain gave the command 'Fruit up.' They fucked guys up real good. Ruben and Youngie weren't around and I didn't want to insult these guys, so I said okay and gave them my name. They wrote it down on a piece of paper and gave me a time and cell number. I figured, what could be the harm of going to a meeting?

"That night I went to the meeting. A member of the FOI stood guard outside the cell and there were seven guys already inside. I knew that was an infraction of prison rules, 'cause you were never supposed to have more than five guys in your cell at any one time. One guy was talking and leading the meeting, and he kept pointing to an easel that was at his side. The pictures were made up of stick figures and were designed to show different historical events and incidents.

"The guy speaking was very intense and well-spoken. He was saying things like, 'The Messenger came to the black man in the wilderness of North America to give them knowledge of themselves and lead them to salvation. The white man purposefully and deceitfully killed off all knowledge of your elders, and now the black man is wandering through the wilderness not knowing a thing about himself or his history.'

"He'd then flip a page on the easel and there'd be a picture of a white man looking like a dog with large teeth, and the next picture was of this same white man with large teeth, but this time he'd be chewing on little black children. Then he'd flip another page and it would show white men raping a black mother and daughter, and the instructor would say, 'This is your grandmother. This is your grandmother being raped. This is what went on under white overseers on black farms all across America.'

"Then he'd say, 'The Messenger was divinely sent to lead the lost and found black man in the wilderness of North America to salvation and freedom. God in the person of Fard Muhammad instructed the Messenger, the Honorable Elijah Muhammad, as to his mission on earth. He was sent to wake up the Asiatic black man and instruct him as to his fullest potential and throw off the white man's shackles that have kept him suppressed and ignorant.'

"For the next hour or two he kept on talking about what the slave master did to us and what the white man had done to the black man in North America. He kept on showing these ugly pictures of black people getting raped and shot and beaten up, their houses burned, and their property destroyed. Pictures of black farmhands having sex with white men while under guard of shotgun-toting guards. I'm telling you, after a while my adrenalin was really pumping. They had me so damn angry, I was ready to attack the first white man I saw. If they would have said, 'We're going rush center and take over the jail,' I would have been there. I would have done it. My head was swimming in anger. I walked out of that cell gritting my teeth, my eyes bulging, and my hands curled up in a tight fist. They had me so fucked up I was gonna jump the first white guy I saw. They were preaching hate and I bought it.

"When I got back to my cell, Youngie and Ruben knew something was up right away. Youngie said, 'Ruben, look at that crazy nigger. Man, did they fuck with his head or what. Butch, you is one sick nigger.'

"Youngie and Ruben had to unhypnotize me. They said, 'Butch, you better watch yourself or you're gonna end up in the hole.' Youngie said the Black Muslims just preach hate and were made up of guys who are gonna be shipped to the penitentiary, guys with long sentences, guys always being thrown in the hole, and guys who are always being watched and under suspicion.

"'Leave those crazy niggers alone,' said Youngie. 'Don't fuck with them. They'll only get you in trouble and ruin your life more than it is already.'

"Youngie was my psychiatrist. He straightened me out. One meeting was enough. I said Salaam Alaikum, nigger. I realized I wasn't about that.

They were teaching hate. They were injecting venom into guys. Fortunately, I had some old heads with me who set me straight. If I hadn't had some experienced brothers watching my back, I may have joined out of fear. A lot of guys joined the NOI because they didn't know anybody in the jail and felt they needed someone to watch their back. A lot of guys were susceptible to that shit 'cause they didn't have the heart to say no when the brothers came fishing for recruits.

"That was the first and last one of their meetings I went to, but it didn't stop them from trying to reel me back into the fold. They figured they got me once, they could do it again. Just about every night they'd come knocking at my cell door. 'Brother Anthony, you gonna join us tonight? Do you wanna receive the words of the Messenger, the Honorable Elijah Muhammad?'

"I always told them I was busy or couldn't make it for some reason or other. It was really getting to be a pain, but I couldn't curse them out and tell them to get lost 'cause that would have been the end of me. They might have rushed me in my cell, and without Ruben and Youngie, I would have been shanked to hell. I knew they were getting irritated that I was always blowing them off, so finally I just told them how I felt. I tried to be diplomatic so they wouldn't take offense, but I had it with them bothering me all the time. A couple of them came to my cell one night and said, 'Brother Anthony, will you be joining us tonight?'

"'Listen, man,' I told them, 'I hope you don't take this the wrong way, but I'm not about that. I won't be coming to any more meetings. I wasn't raised that way. My people were devout Baptists. I was taught to love your neighbor regardless of what color he was. God is love. What you're teaching is nothing what I was taught in church. What you're teaching is hate. I've got nothing against white people.'

"'Listen, brother, all of your problems are due to white people. You're in this here jail because of white people. You need to be educated. You're still running around in the wilderness of your ignorance.'

"'Listen, man,' I replied, 'I'm in here because of the dumb shit I did. And let me tell you something, every time I been hurt it's been because of people with this.' I pointed to the color of the skin on my arm. 'And every time I was in bad shape, every time I needed help, I got it from some white folks. They were the ones who helped me. Not my own people.'

"They looked at me like I was out of my mind. 'You wanna stay dead. You're just an ignorant nigger. Brother, you really are in the wilderness.'

"'That may be,' I said, 'but I ain't coming to any more of your meetings.'

"They never pressed me again to come to a meeting. The Muslims would pass my cell at night as they went up and down the block fishing for new recruits, but they'd walk by my cell without saying a word. I was pretty fortunate I was hooked up. I had some pull in the jail. A lot of tough guys in the criminal world knew me or my family. There were a lot of us from the Village doing time in Holmesburg, and that kept the weight off of me. If I hadn't been connected, the FOI probably would have moved on me. They didn't take it lightly when someone gave them some lip or said something bad about the Messenger. I had just decided I had had enough of them and their mind games and their racist message. I knew I was happiest when I was reading books and playing music. That's what I wanted to do, and that's what I was gonna do while I was locked up."

"He Still Has the Cork in His Ass!"

With the pressure off to join the Nation of Islam, Butch was free to devote more time to his educational pursuits. But even though he now looked forward to reading books, writing letters, and playing the trombone, the oppressive, claustrophobic atmosphere of Holmesburg could still wear an inmate down. Visits from loved ones and optimistic talk of parole from one's attorney could brighten spirits and heighten expectations, but inmates usually fought the swelling tides of pessimism and depression in a variety of ways. One of the most common was making regular trips to the commissary. The purchase of cookies, potato chips, ice cream, and other edible treats, and much sought after personal items like toiletries, could remind one of home and boost one's spirits. But trips to the prison commissary required money. And there was only one way to earn money in Holmesburg—the medical experiments.

Although he had unquestionably suffered through his participation in a patch test and the army's psychotropic drug study, Butch was still susceptible to the jail's siren song—money for a piece of your body. Everyone else in the place, it seemed, was on the tests and making a few bucks. As he put it, "The tests were as routine in the jail as going down to the mess hall for breakfast. That's what the jail was about, testing." As each day passed and he watched others partaking of the various research trials—and the goodies they brought—Butch's adamant opposition to participating in another clinical trial gradually diminished. He didn't like being a human guinea pig, but neither did he like being the only one who wasn't profiting from "what the jail was about."

"Only the Muslims," says Butch, "didn't get on the tests. Everybody else was making money on the tests. It was chump change, but when you're in prison every

8

little bit helps. Blacks, Puerto Ricans, whites, all got on the tests. It was what the jail was about. I sure as hell didn't trust the doctors anymore. They really let me down. I knew they weren't to be trusted. Each time they messed me up I felt like I was suffering in hell. But the tests on H block were an outlet. It was another thing you could do with your time.

"Guys were always telling me what tests they had got on, how much they were making, and what new test the doctors were running. 'Butch, you should get on this test.' Or, 'Butch, they're starting a new test on H block next week and they say it's gonna be paying good money.' I listened, but wanted no parts of them. Gradually, though, I started to think about them again. I needed the money. I told myself maybe it was possible to find one that wouldn't damage me like the others had done. Yeah, a lot of other guys were getting hurt from the tests. Guys were always complaining about rashes and blisters and the scars the burn studies left, but you look at things the way you want. I started to believe there were some medical studies out there that wouldn't be too risky. I just had to be smart and find the right one.

"I asked around, but most of what I was hearing didn't sound safe. There always seemed to be something that made me leery of them. Then I heard one of the guys talking about a diet test that was getting started. He said all you had to do was swallow some diet pills. That was it; just swallow a few pills. It was one of the simplest tests I had heard of and it seemed relatively safe. It wasn't a skin test or some mood-altering test for the army that had messed me up before. I figured I'd look into it a little more.

"I signed up for it when they came down the block looking for volunteers. I listened to what tests the inmate technicians were describing, and when I heard them mention the diet study I put my name down. They told me not to eat anything for breakfast the next morning and I'd be getting a pass to go down to H block. The next morning I got the pass."

Butch wasn't as nervous as he had been the first time he entered H block for a clinical trial. He had been through the drill before. He knew doctors weren't to be trusted and that the element of risk was always there. He was prepared, however, to turn on a dime and walk out if he saw or heard anything that increased his suspicions. He told himself he wasn't the naïve newcomer he had been when he participated in the patch tests months earlier. Butch and about a dozen other men were taken to a lab room on the block, and a University of Pennsylvania test supervisor informed them that they were taking part in a diet study that would require them to take seven pills three times a day. They would have regular meals, except for a special breakfast meal each morning. The study would run twenty-one days and the men would receive $30 when the test was completed.

Butch realized that thirty bucks—a little more than a dollar a day—was chump change compared to what some of the other clinical trials were paying, but $30 looked pretty good when you were broke. "It wasn't much," says Butch, "but it was better than nothing." There was no mention of what the pills actually were, what the doctors were looking for, or what could go wrong—just seven pills, three times a day. They were also told the test was safe.

Skeptical, but reasonably convinced he had found the study with the least threat to his physical and mental health, Butch decided he was in. He needed the money.

The men were weighed, given seven tiny pink pills to swallow, and then escorted to the mess hall. A dozen trays were waiting for them when they arrived. Each contained scrambled eggs, cornflakes, and toast with real butter. The men were delighted—the eggs, bread, and butter all came "from the street"; none of it was the powdered, watered-down, institutional variety that was usually dished out to the prisoners. Compared to the normal prison fare, says Butch, "the breakfasts were a real treat." Only their breakfast meal, however, would be the real deal. Lunches and dinners would be taken as usual with the rest of the inmate population.

The routine remained the same over the next three weeks. Three times each day the same dozen men received passes to go to H block, were given their allotment of pills, and were escorted to the mess hall. Every fourth or fifth day they were weighed on a scale. Two weeks passed without a problem. Just when Butch had convinced himself that he had successfully discovered a relatively safe clinical trial, he came down with a new ailment. He couldn't move his bowels—he was constipated. Though of minor consequence compared to his earlier health maladies, the discomfort worsened with each passing day.

"My stomach was all bloated and I couldn't relieve myself," says Butch. "I'd sit on the toilet for what seemed like hours with no success. I thought about telling the doctors, but I was afraid of being thrown off the test. Guys who developed health problems while on a test were sometimes cut loose. They didn't get paid, and I really needed the money. I didn't want to do anything that was going to jeopardize my participation in the test.

89

"He Still Has the Cork in His Ass!"

That's the reason I never took the shit sauce [Epsom salts] they passed around the jail every morning. Lotta guys had stomach problems from the jail food. All that steamed food was bad for you. Every morning an inmate would come down the block calling out, 'Shit sauce, shit sauce, who needs shit sauce?' Guys would take a cupful if they were having constipation problems. Fortunately, I never had a problem, but now I did. Those pills had messed up my stomach. I was bloated and just passed gas, but couldn't do anything else.

"During the last few days of the test I was really feeling bad. I couldn't wait till it was over so I could take some Epsom salts. Soon as the test was completed and a guard notified me that my money had been placed on the books, I got hold of some Epsom salts. After taking it for two and a half days, it finally worked. But I nearly died in the process. I was on the toilet for a long while. Man, it was terrible. It felt like I was having a baby. My ass was impacted; it felt like concrete had settled in there. All those pills I was taking every day must have messed up my stomach. 'Oh, lord,' I said to myself, 'what the hell is coming out of me?' Sweat was pouring off of me; veins were standing up in my head. It was really terrible. I felt a big knot sticking out of my ass. I was scared to death and didn't know what it was. Really worried, I finally showed Youngie what had popped out of me.

"He took a look and screamed out, 'You got the piles, nigger.'

"'What the fuck are piles?' I asked him.

"'Your ass has turned inside out.'

"'Oh fuck, why does everything have to happen to me?'

"Youngie said I should take my sick ass over to the U of P doctors and have them fix me up. Their test messed me up, so now it was their job to fix me. I couldn't believe it: once again I was forced to go back to H block and have them no-good doctors fix me up after they had ruined me. I could hardly walk with that thing sticking out of me. The block guard wouldn't give me a pass to go to H block. He said my test was over. Even with the way I looked, it took me a while to convince him I needed to see the doctors. He finally gave me a pass, but when I got to H block they wouldn't let me on the block. I told them it was an emergency and I needed to see a doctor. They kept on saying the experiment I was assigned to was over and the only doctor I could see was the doctor who ran my test. I asked when he was coming in, but they didn't know when he'd be returning. I told them I was in bad shape and needed help. It didn't make any difference to them. They kept on saying the same thing. My test was over and the only doctor who would look at me was the one who ran the experiment. But then they'd say they didn't know when he would be in again.

"I was ready to kill somebody. I was bent over in pain and all those doctors on H block wouldn't even look at me. Wouldn't even let me on the block. I was furious, but I was in bad shape and needed help.

"Back in my cell, Youngie said, 'Fuck those Penn doctors. They ain't no goddamn good anyway. Put your name down for sick call and see one of the regular prison doctors. Somebody there will take care of you.'

"I got the block guard to write me out a pass, but instead of going to the regular prison hospital on C block they told me to go over to H block. They said the prison doctor was using the U of P experimentation block because there was more room over there to examine guys. I had to wait a while till it was my turn. Just trying to sit was painful, so I stood the entire time. It took almost two hours. Finally they called my name and I got to see a doctor. I told him I needed some Preparation H or something even stronger than that.

"'What's your problem?' he asked.

"I told him what happened to me on the toilet.

"'Okay,' he said, 'drop your pants.'

"Just hearing that made me feel uncomfortable because of all the ass-hole bandits running around the jail, but I was in desperate need of help. So I did it."

"'Jesus Christ,' the doctor shouted, 'they're beautiful.'

"I thought he was making fun of me, but all I said was, 'Can I now have some Preparation H?'

"'Fella, let me tell you something,' said the doctor. 'You've got a serious problem. You need a hell of a lot more than Preparation H.'

"'Like what?' I asked him.

"'You're gonna need surgery.'

"My heart dropped. I said, 'Surgery? What kind of surgery?'

"'Those hemorrhoids are going to have to be cut and burned.'

"'Oh no.'

"'Oh yes,' said the doctor. 'And I'm not even sure that once we perform surgery they won't return sometime in the future. I'm going to schedule you for a hemorrhoid operation at PGH [Philadelphia General Hospital] tomorrow. Get your belongings together tonight and you'll get a medical pass in the morning.'

"He Still Has the Cork in His Ass!"

After being given some pills to ease the pain, Butch slowly limped off H block and went back to his cell block. Every step was painful. Butch imagined everyone in the jail had his eyes on him. Depressed and angry, he couldn't believe that once again the doctors and their experiments had wrecked his health. Now he was facing surgery in a hospital. He tried to consider the bright side; he'd be getting out of Holmesburg for a short time, and maybe even get some quality time with Laura while he was recovering. But the physical discomfort and specter of surgery destroyed the comforting illusion. All he could think of was that he was damaged goods again.

After a sleepless night, Butch slowly gathered his belongings. Toiletries, underwear, and a few other odds and ends were thrown into a paper bag. His cell mates tried to cheer him up by saying he'd be getting better food down at PGH, clean sheets, and long contact visits with his wife. Then a block worker called out his name and he was handed his pass. He hugged Youngie and Ruben, forced a smile, and said, "I'll be seeing you niggers in a couple weeks."

At center control in Holmesburg's large rotunda Butch joined the other men scheduled for surgery at PGH. When all nine men had gathered, a white-shirted lieutenant came over to take the men to the receiving room and out of the jail. To Butch's surprise, however, he and two other men were separated from the rest of the group. They were then quickly escorted to the prison hospital on C block.

"Wait a second," said Butch, "I'm supposed to be going to PGH for an operation."

"Not today," said the officer. "You're going to the back of C block and the prison hospital."

"No, no," Butch protested, "I'm scheduled for surgery down at PGH."

"Listen, Anthony," said the white-shirted officer firmly, "we got orders for you to go to C block. If the doctors want to change it, that's up to them. Until then you're going to C block."

Confused, but aware that further objections would be of no use, Butch was taken to the prison hospital, a makeshift collection of small rooms and wards that had been added onto the facility after its construction in the 1890s. The other two inmates, both Puerto Ricans, were speaking Spanish and seemed as perplexed as he. Within minutes an inmate medical assistant walked in and told the men to disrobe and put on the hospital gowns he handed them. He then laid a blanket on the floor and told Butch to get down on his hands and knees.

Surprised by the request, Butch inquired, "Why do you want me on my hands and knees?"

"I'm gonna shave your rectum," said the inmate medical assistant matter-of-factly.

"You're gonna what?" bellowed Butch.

"I gotta shave your ass if you're gonna have surgery."

"Oh my God," replied Butch.

"C'mon, get down here," said the inmate, who was already down on one knee and putting a blade in the safety razor. "Believe me, this ain't as bad as what the doctor is gonna do to you."

Always preoccupied with the fear of being placed in a sexually compromising position while incarcerated, Butch was further mortified by having to be spread out on a musty army blanket and having his buttocks shaved by another inmate, and one who was probably a homosexual at that. He was already extremely sensitive because of the protruding hemorrhoid, and each stroke of the razor caused him to flinch and reflect on what he had done to deserve such a painful and embarrassing ordeal. His fear and disillusionment mounted as both Puerto Rican inmates preceded him into surgery and he apprehensively waited his turn on a hospital bed to face the knife.

93

"What the hell did I do to deserve this?" Butch kept saying to himself. Why, every time he got on one of the prison tests, did something go radically wrong and burden him with some serious medical malady? The more he thought about it, the more his strict Baptist upbringing kicked in. God, no doubt, was punishing him for something terrible he had done. All those hellfire-and-brimstone sermons he had heard in church as a child came crashing back on him. He was certain that God was punishing him for all the wrongs he had committed over the years. Disrespecting his parents, playing hooky from school, getting drunk on cheap wine, not supporting his wife and child properly, and the drugs, always the drugs—these were the reasons for his descent into hell.

That's what jail had become for Edward "Butch" Anthony, hell on earth. He had been forewarned what to expect at Holmesburg, but the actual reality of it, and the toll it had taken on his health and psyche, were totally unexpected. The entire place was crazy. Butch understood that people who broke the law or harmed others should be separated from society and placed in a secure facility where they could do no further harm. But Holmesburg was a madhouse. The violence was pervasive, sexual assaults were routine, and religious zealots were engaged in a constant feeding frenzy. And if that wasn't bad enough, the bizarre medical experiments were the clincher. Things he had never conceived of were routinely being done to people. "How did I get in this place?" he kept asking himself.

"Anthony. Edward Anthony, your turn."

The female voice was pleasant enough, but he had learned to fear that the mellifluous tones emanating from this area of the prison were certain to lead sheep to the slaughter. "C'mon, it's your turn," said the nurse, leading him into the small, primitive operating room. The air was thick with disinfectant. A rather small, rotund man in a white lab coat had his back turned to him, while two inmate assistants, both husky six-footers, stood on the side and eyed him with the interest of factory meat cutters spying another side of beef.

"Okay, Anthony," said the doctor, who reminded Butch of the Dr. Magoo comic strip character. "Take off the dressing gown. Up on the table and on your stomach."

Butch lay down on the table and saw the doctor pick up a long metal probe with an egg-shaped contraption at one end.

"This will be a little painful, but it will stop soon," said the doctor as he applied an oily lubricant to the probe.

Just as he plunged it into Butch's rectum, the two inmates positioned themselves above Butch and grabbed his wrists. Butch took a deep breath and could feel the probe enter him and smack up against his backbone. Then he could feel the doctor do something with the handle so that the probe's prongs opened up inside him. There were a couple of quick twists, and then Butch nearly cleared the table as the doctor pulled on the probe and turned his rectum inside out.

Butch tried to catch his breath and stop hyperventilating as beads of sweat multiplied on his forehead. He then spied the doctor with a huge syringe that appeared to contain a mixture of liquid and rock candy. Butch prayed it was Novocain or some other powerful painkiller. He then felt a series of injections in a clockwise direction starting with the tip of his spine. The final injection was in the hemorrhoid itself, causing Butch to emit a string of curses and try to thrust himself off the table.

"Did you see that fuck?" said the doctor of the hemorrhoid's reaction to the injection. The inmates nodded, but were too busy angling themselves for better leverage as Butch squirmed and screamed to be released.

Sentenced To Science

"Get the fuck off me, you dirty muthafuckers," Butch cried out. "You're tryin' to kill me. Get the hell off of me or I'll kill you, you dirty bastards."

The pain was excruciating, and now Butch could feel himself being cut. The pain was so clear, it was if he hadn't received any anesthetic at all. He was hollering at the top of his lungs, so loudly, in fact, that the nurse who had been caring for the two Puerto Rican inmates in an adjoining room came running in to see what all the commotion was about.

"I felt every fucking thing they were doing," recalls Butch. "It was incredibly painful. I wanted to kill the doctor. I wanted to kill him before he killed me. I would have, too, if those damn niggers hadn't been sitting on my shoulders and legs holding me down. Even with the five shots of Novocain I could still feel everything that was going on. I was screaming so loud the nurse came rushing in and started wiping a sponge across my brow to soak up the balls of sweat that were forming. 'It'll all be over soon,' she kept on saying. 'The doctor is almost done.'

"All I knew was that this fat little Dr. Magoo was tryin' to kill me and I was suffering the worst pain of my life. I kept on cursing him and tried to get at him, but these big niggers were holding me down. I couldn't understand why the Puerto Rican dudes went through the operation with hardly a whimper and I was screaming my head off. Why did everything have to happen to me?"

Soon the smell of burning flesh filled the room as the doctor cauterized the wound left from the severed hemorrhoid. Butch, still cursing and pleading to be released, was writhing and churning on the table like a bucking stallion. Through sweat-soaked eyes, he next saw the doctor lubricate another long metal probe and attach half a dozen large gauze pads to one end. Then he felt the probe inserted into his rectum.

"Almost done," said the doctor.

Butch didn't believe him for a second. The white-cloaked physician had caused him the worst pain he had ever endured. Doctors weren't to be trusted, Holmesburg had taught him that. They weren't healers; they were sadists. Butch, and others like him, were just meat on the hoof. Subhumans who had value only as test subjects. Never would he trust a doctor again.

The doctor continued to pack the gaping wound and then covered it with a Kotex sanitary napkin. Butch heard the doctor say, "You're done, Anthony. You can get up now." The inmates released their grip on Butch's arms and legs, and the last thing he recalls seeing were their fingerprints

"He Still Has the Cork in His Ass!"

on his wrists and forearms. As he raised himself off the operating table, he passed out and had to be carried to his hospital bed.

"I don't know how long I was unconscious," recalls Butch, "but when I came to, the pain was excruciating. I was in a bed in the hospital ward and the pain was terrible. It felt like somebody had shoved a red-hot pipe up my ass. At first I was just moaning, but I soon started screaming, 'What did you motherfuckers do to me? Gimme something for the pain, you hear? Gimme something to kill the pain.' There were a few other guys in the hospital ward, and they were looking at me like I was crazy, but I didn't give a shit. I was dying. The pain was awful."

Finally, a nurse came over to tend to the complaining patient. As she started to fluff his pillow she asked, "What seems to be the problem?"

"My ass is on fire," barked Butch. "I need something for the pain. Please give me something quick. I can't take this pain any longer."

"Okay," said the nurse. "Let me see what your chart says."

Butch prayed she'd return with something strong. He knew he'd never be able to last without some kind of painkiller. In addition to the pain, his heart was beating so fast he feared he'd have a heart attack. Even the slightest movement seemed to heighten his discomfort. When the nurse didn't return, Butch began to scream for help once again. The other patients took notice, but most turned over in their beds and wrapped their pillows around their ears. When the nurse returned she displayed a frown and said, "I'm sorry Mr. Anthony, but you have drugs on your record. We can't give you any pain medication."

"You what?" replied Butch in disbelief.

"You have drugs on your prison record," repeated the nurse. "We have a policy that prevents us from . . ."

"Listen, bitch," Butch interrupted, "you better get me something for this pain or I'm gonna tear this fucking place apart. You hear me? I'm gonna kill somebody. You people rip the shit out of my ass and then gonna tell me I can't have any goddamn Bufferin. Now you better come back here with something strong to stop this pain or I'm gonna get out of this bed and do some damage."

Butch managed to prop himself up on his elbows and act as if he was about to carry out his threat. Properly sensitized to the surly patient's concerns, the nurse quickly ran off to the nurse's station. When she returned she was carrying four pills in a paper cup—two Darvocet and two other pain capsules that Butch swallowed immediately. Within minutes Butch was asleep, but each time he awoke, the pain and the cries for medication were renewed. The next day Butch expected to see a doctor, but none came. A nurse would periodically stop by his bed, but she had very little information to offer. Butch was constantly seeking additional medication from her. He wondered why he was cursed with such pain and discomfort while the Puerto Rican boys who had been operated on seemed to be in fine spirits and spent most of each day playing cards. "Why the hell am I screaming in bed and hollering for help," Butch would ask himself, "when they're moving around and playing cards?" He never received a satisfactory answer.

The second day, his discomfort increased. Being told that no physician was expected to examine him did not allay his concerns. Once again he had been abandoned. He felt like he had to move his bowels, but he feared what would happen. His rectum was still packed with medical dressing and gauze pads and he still hadn't received any directions from the doctor. Was he supposed to remove the dressing from the wound himself, or was he supposed to wait for the doctor to examine him? As was the custom at Holmesburg, the doctors never told you anything. And there were always more than enough reasons to assume that the less contact you had with medical people, the better.

While Butch was mulling over what he should do, another drama was being played out in the prison hospital. An inmate who had suffered a bad reaction to one of the army's psychotropic drug studies had locked himself in the bathroom. He had been brought to the block after acting bizarrely and claiming to see birds flying through the walls of his cell. Brought to the OBS unit on C block, he had managed to lock himself in the bathroom. Several hours went by. Guards finally considered breaking the door down and rushing the hallucinatory prisoner, when they conceived of a less violent plan. They seduced the inmate into opening the door by telling him they had brought birdseed and cages for the birds. He was quickly subdued and placed in a straitjacket. Though the affair seemed to have ended well enough, Butch had little difficulty comprehending the moral of the story— doctors and their damn experiments can mess you up.

With the bathroom open for use again, Butch decided it was now time for him to take some action. He slowly gathered himself up and made it over to one of the bathroom toilets. If it were feasible, he'd pull the packing out of his rectum and try to defecate. It didn't take long, however, to recognize that scenario as highly improbable. Massive amounts of blood had coagulated around his anus, locking the bandages in place like a well-fortified levee. Not only weren't the bandages and gauze pads coming out, Butch also told himself, "ain't nothing coming through this asshole. I'm just gonna be having liquids until a doctor fixes me up."

By the third day, Butch was sure the prison's plan was to torture him to death. He still hadn't seen a doctor, much less the surgeon who had operated on him. The packing was still intact, his stomach was bloated, he hadn't defecated in more than three days, and the pain was still as excruciating as ever. His pleas for painkillers had kept the other inmates in the hospital awake around the clock and placed a perpetual frown on the faces of the meager nursing staff.

Finally, on the evening of the third day, a doctor appeared. A nurse briefed him on the state of the ward saying, "Everything is fine except for this one patient. He's still in pain and is constantly screaming and hollering for pain medication. We don't know what to do with him."

"Okay," said the doctor, "let's take a look at him."

The doctor approached Butch's bed and said, "What seems to be the problem, Mr. Anthony?"

"Doc, I'm in bad shape. You gotta do something for me."

"All right. Turn over and let me take a look."

Butch gingerly turned on his stomach and the doctor spread his butt checks apart. "No wonder," cried the doctor, "he still has the cork in his ass!"

Butch didn't need the doctor to explain what had happened. He knew immediately that the medical staff had forgotten to remove the packing from his rectum. Because he had passed out after the surgery, the doctor had never instructed him as to the proper postoperative care he required. He was never told he would need to take sitz baths to loosen the blood-soaked bandages, what to eat and not eat, and what to expect the first time he moved his bowels. The fact that the Puerto Rican patients only spoke Spanish only added to the mystery.

"Hold on," said the doctor, "this'll just take a second."

Suddenly, with only those few words of warning, the doctor ripped the cork, gauze pads, and adhesive tape out of Butch's rectum. As a spray of blood, ripped stitches, moist scabs, and stained medical dressing flew across the room, Butch grabbed the bed, then bounced upward as if shot from a cannon. No proper warning, no sitz bath, no nothing—just the doctor yanking the solidly implanted, three-day-old packing out of the patient's rectum. In addition to the sharp pain, a thought shot through

Butch's brain—he was being tortured by the doctors for some serious sin he had committed. This was definitely retribution.

To add insult to injury, Butch would soon discover that proper aftercare was an illusion at Holmesburg; he was being sent back to his own block immediately. Butch would have bet anything that the renewed bleeding from the stitches being abruptly pulled apart would have necessitated another day or two in the hospital ward, but he was mistaken. After the doctor cleaned the wound and covered it with a woman's sanitary napkin, the patient was sent back to population.

"I couldn't believe they were sending me back to the block," recalls Anthony. "I was in bad shape and could hardly walk. I had to hold on to the wall to take a step. They messed me up after surgery, put me in additional pain, and when they find out their mistake, they snatch the packing out of me like I was a dog and send me back to my dirty, stinkin' cell block. They weren't doctors, they were sadists."

Butch ambulated as best he could through Holmesburg's rotunda toward his cell. Weak and feeling faint, he held on to the wall for stability the entire time. Butch was fortunate to have been spotted by his cell mates, Youngie and Ruben, who were on their way to the mess hall for dinner. The men got out of line and helped carry Butch back to their cell. They couldn't help but notice a bloody stain forming in the seat of his pants. Once they had gently laid Butch down on his bunk, Youngie took a good look at his cell mate. He slowly shook his head in disbelief and said, "You look terrible, man. What the hell did they do to you?"

"They're trying to kill me," whispered Butch. "Those motherfuckers are trying to kill me."

99

"Those Doctors Ain't Interested in You"

A damp, unsanitary Holmesburg cell block was no place to recover from surgery or severe illness. Skin, respiratory, and sexually transmitted diseases were rampant, and relapses were so commonplace that there was a revolving door relationship between the city's largest prison in Northeast Philadelphia and Philadelphia General Hospital, the financially strapped city hospital in West Philadelphia. Both underfunded and understaffed facilities tended to the needs of the city's poor and downtrodden. As one of the "great unwashed"—as some called the mentally deficient, morally challenged, and economically deprived—that inhabited one or the other of the institutions, Butch spent an inordinate amount of time in his cell dwelling on his wretched circumstances. As the hours and days passed without the proper medical guidance, aftercare treatment, and pain medication, he couldn't help but reflect on his life, the insensitivity of doctors, and society in general. The prison's so-called healers received particular attention.

He knew that his actions alone had culminated in a prison sentence, but was it because he was in jail that the doctors—a profession he had been brought up to respect and admire—were treating him in such a cavalier manner? "Is it because I'm a criminal that the doctors are acting this way?" he'd ask his cell mates. "Or is it because I'm a poor, uneducated black man that they won't give me the treatment and care I need?"

"I don't know, Butch," replied Youngie, "but you always seem to get fucked up. I don't know what it is with you."

"It's almost like they see me coming and say, 'We're gonna teach Edward Anthony a lesson.'"

"You gotta be like me," boasted Youngie. "You gotta be a little more selective as to what you get involved with. Some of those tests are nasty, but a lot of them are okay."

9

Shaking his head in disagreement, Butch knew he had been as scrupulous as possible in deciding what tests to get on. He looked for those trials that presented the least risk of injury. They always paid the least, but the tradeoff was greater confidence that he wouldn't be harmed. Even that didn't work, however. He was still getting "fucked up."

Others on the block were less forgiving than Butch's cell mate. Mack, a bodybuilder Butch knew from Edison High School, was damaged in one of the patch tests and never participated in another. He'd visit Butch in his cell and tell him, "I told you to stay off those tests. You remember when you had to help me get those patches and chemicals off my back 'cause I was being burned so bad. I'm still carrying the scars from that shit. You gotta be a fool to keep going back. Fuck those tests. Those doctors ain't interested in you."

"It's money, man," Youngie would occasionally interject. "You want commissary, don't you?"

"Not if they're gonna fuck me up," Mack shot back. "Those doctors ain't gonna mess with this nigger again, commissary or no commissary. Let them find some other dumb motherfucker to screw around with."

Pathetically slow already, Butch's recovery hit an additional snag when he was thrown in the hole for ten days. The punishment, which Butch felt was clearly unwarranted, did further harm to his already fragile mental and physical health. The penalty arose when Butch was caught hanging around the corridor leading to band room. The officer who wrote him up considered Butch a malingerer who refused to work. In his view, the inmate had time for jazz and shooting the breeze with other deadbeats, but not for his required prison chores. He was unimpressed by Butch's hemorrhoid surgery and its aftermath and expected him, after a reasonable amount of time, to be back to work at his job in the knit shop.

For Butch, being thrown in the hole was the last straw. He couldn't fathom things getting any worse. A "torn-up asshole" thanks to insensitive doctors and a lousy experiment, and now this, ten days in a strip cell. It was torture, plain and simple. Butch told the guard and the "kangaroo court" that sentenced him what had transpired, but it was like talking to the wall. Because of his absence during and after surgery, band members had informed him that if he wasn't going to participate in the prison music program, he should return the trombone he had borrowed. He didn't want to part with the horn, but he realized that the surgery had taken a lot out of him and that he was in no mood to play the instrument. When he went to return it, he heard the full band practicing a piece and decided to wait outside the room until they were finished. He well knew the distraction it caused when someone entered the band room while musicians were concentrating on a new score. His diplomacy resulted in his second stretch in the hole.

"Here I go again," said Butch of his feelings at the time. "It was crazy shit. No clothes, one meal a day, no medication for my sick ass. It was torture. The pain and the itching were terrible. Then this pus started to come out of me, so I knew it had become infected. Every time I had to defecate I was worried I was getting the open wound infected. But what can I do? I'm in the hole. When I would tell the guards I gotta see a doctor, they just slammed the door in my face and the cell went black.

"I got so frustrated I started to compose a letter in my head. I was planning on sending it to the judge that had originally sentenced me. I had no paper or pencil or anything else in the hole to write with so I made it up and memorized the whole thing. I added a little each day. I told him I was given time for a crime I did. I told him I could live with that, but all the other shit was uncalled for. All the crazy sex and extreme violence in the jail was over the top. And worst of all were the medical experiments. I told him people were gettin' killed and mentally fucked up on those tests. I told him how I had been messed up on the patch test, the army test, and the diet study. I described how I hadn't even recovered from hemorrhoid surgery when they threw me in the hole, and now my rectum was infected. I told him it was bad enough being sentenced to serve time, without having to be sentenced to science as well. I thought it was a pretty good letter, but I couldn't really send it. It was all in my head."

103

There is a very good chance that Butch would have composed the letter on paper and mailed it, but once he was released from the hole he had one thing on his mind—getting healthy. His lengthy isolation in primitive quarters and lack of medication had aggravated his condition. Repeated visits to the Holmesburg hospital ward and getting the right treatment were now his paramount concern.

Butch's slow recovery from surgery eventually caused a rift between the prison's medical staff and the University of Pennsylvania's research program. Tired of dealing with Butch's constant requests for gauze pads, sanitary napkins, medicinal lubricants, and pain medication, the city prison doctors sought the assistance of the H block researchers to supply some of the needed items. Initially, the Penn physicians disowned any responsibility for inmate Anthony's medical troubles, arguing that they were unaware of any complications resulting from his participation in one of their clinical trials. Prison doctors, well acquainted with his case by now, replied that Edward Anthony's hemorrhoid surgery was a direct result of his participation in a diet study. Though the Penn doctors were reluctant to accept that argument, the research unit eventually complied and produced stronger medication and effective salves and ointments that were markedly better than what he had been receiving.

"The regular jail medication was shit," says Butch. "Days were going by and I wasn't getting any better. I couldn't go to work or partake of anything else in the jail. It was really cruel. My faith in doctors was shot. I looked at what they did to me and some other guys with medical problems and then at what they didn't do for guys who needed help, and said, 'These doctors are sadists.' After three or four weeks of this, I finally got the H block medication and started to heal. They gave me a tube of medication that inserted into a device that I placed in my rectum. It must have been strong, because I finally started to get well."

Though his physical health gradually improved, Butch's psyche had apparently suffered a more severe wound. He socialized with other inmates less frequently now and spent an inordinate amount of time in his cell. He became withdrawn and solitary.

"I didn't trust anybody," recalls Butch. "I didn't trust the doctors, the guards, the inmates. I just wanted to be left alone. I didn't even go down to the band room that often. I just practiced on my own in the cell when I could borrow a horn, and I wasn't even doing much of that anymore. That last test and the problems it caused really took a lot out of me. It even killed my interest in music."

Butch's behavior eventually began to irritate his cell mates, especially Youngie. An old head with many prison years under his belt, Youngie was a carefree operator who knew how to maneuver in the jail, get over on people, and create novel ways to enhance his prison income. A jailhouse Bobby Fischer on the chessboard and an accomplished Lothario in the personals, he managed to talk several women on the West Coast into sending him money. Informed, upbeat, and always looking for the next score, he grew bored with Butch's depression. Yeah, Butch had been beat up in the tests, but his lousy attitude was sucking the air out of the cell. Youngie would invite members of his crew back to his cell for periodic bridge games and bullshit sessions, and Butch would just lie on his bed and stare into space. It was unnerving. He expected Butch to snap out of it. Their growing disenchantment with each other finally reached the boiling point.

"Youngie would always be telling me, 'Don't lay around, man. You're too goddamn reclusive. You're acting like an old man. Get up and do something.' It was really starting to piss me off. I didn't feel like being a damn party animal. The prison, the experiments, the lousy doctors had wrecked me. I didn't trust anybody, not the correctional officers, not the doctors, not the social workers, no one. I just wanted to be left alone, but Youngie was always pushing me to hang with this crowd or be part of this group or try this test and start making some money. I had finally had it with him.

"One day we were getting into it. He was peppering me with that dumb shit that I didn't want to hang out. That he and his crew were lively, upbeat guys, and I was puttin' the brakes on them. He then says, 'You know, Butch, maybe you just need to move the hell out of here.' I told him, 'I'd be glad to move outta here, motherfucker.'

"We nearly came to blows, but it woulda been a long day in hell before that skinny-assed motherfucker would ever beat one of Joseph Anthony's children. Besides, Youngie was afraid of me. Ever since that army experiment, Youngie thought I was nuts. I'd be laughing and talking at inappropriate times while that shit was in my system. He couldn't forget how I acted. He was scared of me. I had celled with him over a year and needed a change anyway.

"I talked to the block guard and he let me move in with Merv, one of the guys from the band who played the baritone sax and was really into music. Soon after, Joe, a piano player, celled up with us. We got along well and were always talking music, technique, and practicing with our instruments. We'd spend hours talking about Monk, Getz, Mingus, and Bill Evans. Those guys really got me back into music again."

During the next couple of months Butch's attitude and overall health improved. He was back at work in the tailor shop, practicing with the band, and counting the days until his release. Money was still an issue, but he had had enough of the medical experiments. Guys would suggest one or the other of the tests to him as a way to make some quick money, but he turned them down cold. He knew they were dangerous and that it was a cruel joke to think you could find one that was guaranteed not to hurt you. With his luck, he realized that even a simple soap test or aspirin study would probably leave him injured and hospitalized. The tests were a crapshoot, and Butch had repeatedly proved himself a stone-cold loser.

Suddenly, however, his relatively peaceful routine was shattered. He was called down to center one morning before work and informed that he was being transferred to the "Creek." The institution, just a stone's throw from Holmesburg, nestled at the confluence of the Delaware River and Penny-pack Creek, was short of laundry workers, and Butch, along with a dozen others, were assigned to be the replacements. Not sure whether to be happy or sad, Butch knew he had fewer than six months' time left to serve, and maybe this would take him a step closer to home. Holmesburg was the roughest jail in the city, and he wouldn't miss the turmoil, but he had grown accustomed to his new cell mates and enjoyed the musically supportive atmosphere they had established. The Creek, however, offered the prospect of a safer environment—less violence and less scientific research.

Another spoke-and-wheel facility built in the 1920s, the House of Correction, as it was formally called, actually dated to the 1880s, when prisoners were moved by barge up and down the Delaware to face court proceedings about ten miles away in Philadelphia City Hall. Although the jail's demographic makeup in terms of race, class, and population capacity was quite similar to Holmesburg's, it tended to hold inmates who were less violent and facing less serious charges. From an inmate's perspective, it had a few other appealing characteristics—the Creek held women, and it wasn't surrounded by an ominous thirty-five-foot wall. For Butch, it was a "breath of fresh air."

"I liked the House of Correction better," says Butch of his new accommodations. "There was a freer atmosphere there. You could see the ships and boats on the river, cars on the highway, and people coming for visits. You could see women and spend time looking at the girls who were locked on G wing. Some of them were pretty cute, but others looked like weightlifters. They had muscles like Steve Reeves, and it looked like a few of those girls could break a motherfucker's back.

"There was less pressure in the Creek, which meant fewer fights. They had more activities and programs for guys to get involved with. There were lots of teachers to help you get an education and your GED diploma, more yard time, and swag sandwiches were easier to get ahold of. It was a playhouse compared to the Burg."

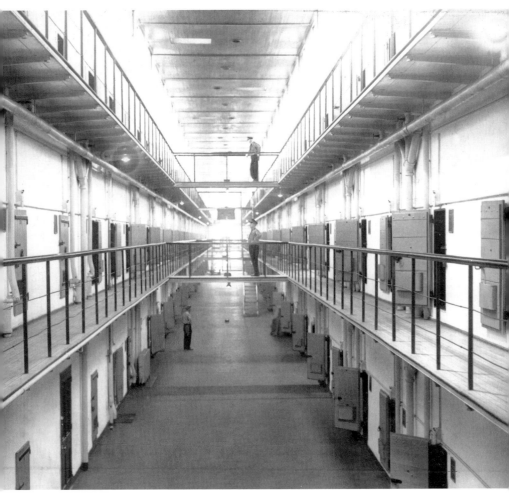

Eddie Anthony's first taste of prison life was Moyamensing Prison, a pre—Civil War relic constructed in the 1830s. "Moko," as the aging facility was commonly called, impressed Anthony with its "wooden floors, rats as large as cats" and its menacing clientele.

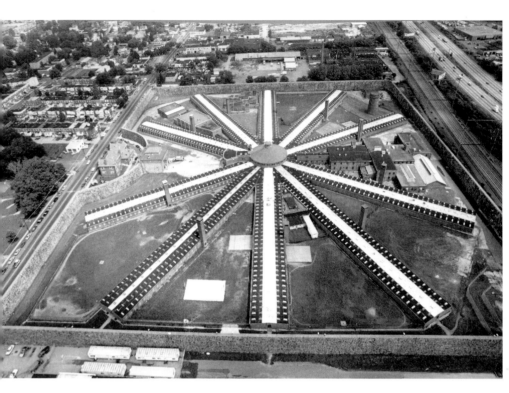

Constructed in the traditional spoke-and-wheel design favored by penal architects in the nineteenth century, Holmesburg quickly developed a reputation for "hardness" as it became home to Philadelphia's most violent offenders.

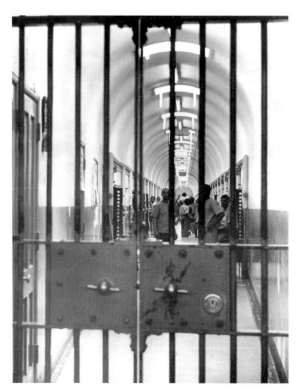

Built in the 1890s, Holmesburg Prison was a large big-city jail that contained an assortment of social miscreants and dangerous criminals. Gang wars, "blanket parties," and bizarre medical experiments characterized life on Holmesburg's cell blocks.

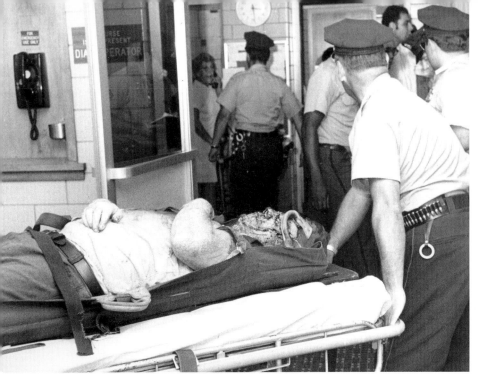

Holmesburg had its share of nasty prison riots over the years. The July 4th, 1970, riot was particularly grim. Many considered the bloody skirmish an outright race riot that targeted whites for retribution.

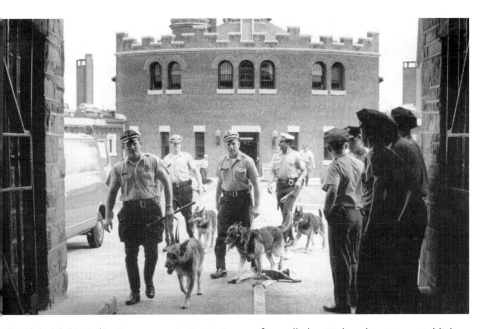

The Philadelphia Police Department's K-9 Unit was often called to Holmesburg to reestablish order. Most Philly cops couldn't imagine how prison guards worked the ever-dangerous cell blocks without anything more than a pencil and a whistle.

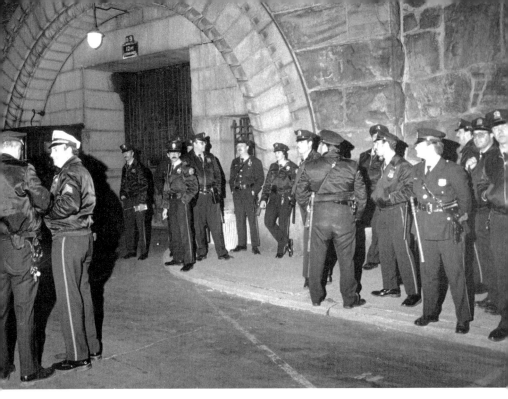

The assembling of Philadelphia police outside the walls of Holmesburg was not an unusual occurrence. Riots, cell-block gang wars, and escapes often drew an emergency response.

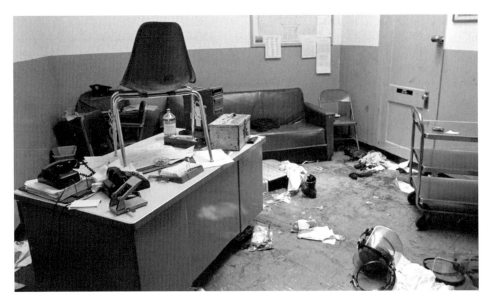

The bloody, disheveled office where Warden Curran and Deputy Warden Fromhold were stabbed to death in 1973. The brutal murders solidified Holmesburg's reputation as one of the nation's most violent urban jails.

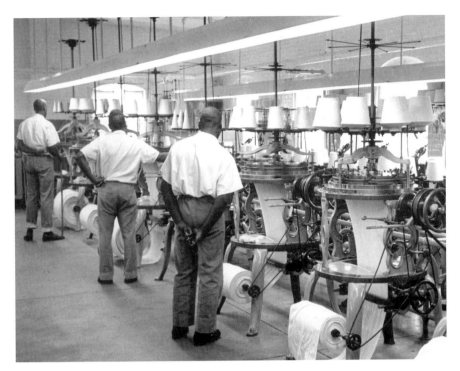

If a Holmesburg inmate was fortunate enough to get a job, he was likely to make no more than 25 cents a day. Butch Anthony occasionally worked in the prison's knit shop making clothes for prisoners.

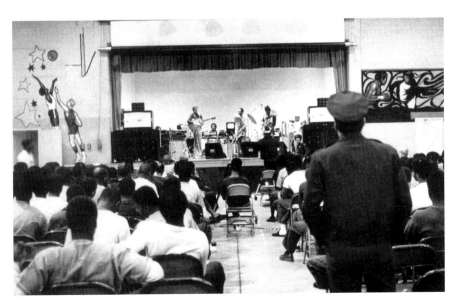

Anthony discovered that music was one of the few ways to relieve stress while serving time in the Philly jails. Although a musical novice, he practiced for hours and enjoyed spending time with musicians who were serious about their craft.

Yusef's older brother Joe Anthony was a large, barrel-chested pugilist who put on boxing exhibitions with heavyweight champion Joe Lewis for American troops during World War II. Joe is pictured here with his mother and wife, Rose. (family photo)

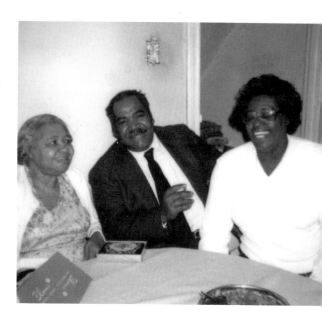

Brother Wilbert was a stable force in the Anthony household and was regularly forced to keep a close watch on his younger, drug-prone sibling. (family photo)

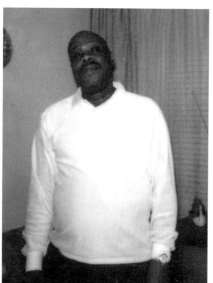

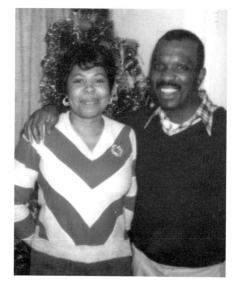

Sister Alease (pictured here with her husband, Jerry) was pressed into action on numerous occasions when her brother ran afoul of the law or his health was endangered. (family photo)

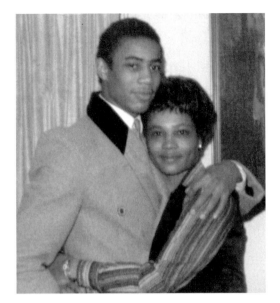

Laura, Yusef's first wife, was forced to contend with her husband's personal insecurities, drug addiction, and repeated incarcerations. She is pictured here with her son, Edward Jr. (family photo)

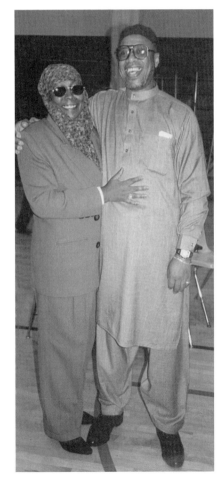

Jemillah and Yusef Anthony have weathered both personal and physical storms over the years. Their commitment to each other and their religious faith have allowed them to endure and survive. (family photo)

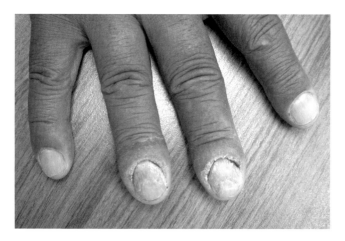

After many years of both care and embarrassment, Yusef's fingernails have begun to look almost normal again. At one time resembling half-inch-thick ugly claws, they had been deformed after his hands had "swelled to the size of 8-ounce boxing gloves." (photo: George Holmes)

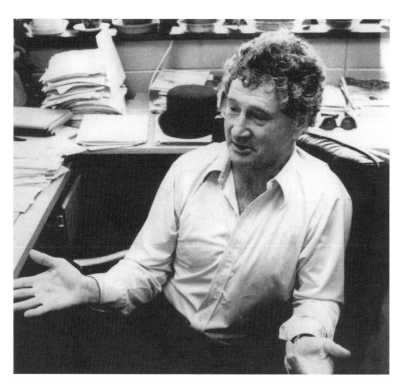

Albert M. Kligman was one of America's most famous dermatologists during the second half of the twentieth century. Described as "brilliant," "creative," and a "wonderful raconteur," he was also quite comfortable using institutionalized children, prisoners, and senior citizens as research material.

Assigned to the laundry, Butch manned three noisy machines that in quick succession pressed the arms, the collars and shoulders, the back and front, and finally folded inmates' shirts. It was a laborious, physically taxing job, but when he got a rhythm going Butch considered it a form of therapy. Not afraid of hard work, he enjoyed the labor. In fact, his enthusiasm for the work nearly resulted in a physical confrontation with co-workers.

"I got into an argument with Brooks, an old head who said I was working too fast. He told me to slow down. When I didn't, he called me an Uncle Tom 'cause I was working so hard for the man. He said I was making him and the other guys look bad. I said, 'Fuck you, I'm gonna work the way I wanna work.' I said, 'Fuck all of you.' That laundry work was a release for me."

Back in his cell on F1 at night, Butch quickly adapted to the pastime of choice among the prison workers—getting high on glue after dinner. Because the grounds of the House of Correction contained a number of maintenance facilities for the upkeep of the city's three prisons, inmate workers were able to get their hands on numerous contraband items. Glue from the wood shop was one of them. Smuggled into the prison inside baby food jars or other containers, the inmates would soak a rag in glue, place it in a paper or plastic bag, and then start huffing. The desired effect was attained fairly quickly, and some even compared it to a marijuana high. With no televisions on the block at that time and nothing comparable to Holmesburg's music program to occupy his time, Butch devoted his nights to sticking his head inside fume-filled paper bags.

It was while Butch was in one of these glue-induced stupors that he made a shocking decision—he'd participate in another experiment.

Though he certainly could have used the few bucks he would have earned, Butch had entirely lost interest in the medical studies. Since the last diet study at Holmesburg, he hadn't been tempted to enter another trial. He knew better than anyone how the tests had damaged his physical and mental health. Fortunately, the University of Pennsylvania research program at the House of Correction was a scaled-down version of what was taking place inside the walls of Holmesburg. He was glad of that—the less visibility and prominence, the less temptation.

The temptation factor was ratcheted up considerably, however, when he heard that the pills provided in one drug study acted like a soothing narcotic. Edward "Butch" Anthony, the incontrovertible drug addict, was all ears.

107

"We were huffing away one night, when one of the guys said, 'Between the glue and the sleeping pills the U of P doctors are givin' me in this drug study, I'm the most mellowed-out motherfucker in this here jail.' I asked him what he was talking about and he told us the Penn doctors were doing some sleep studies in the jail, and the drugs they were givin' out were just like Valium. They just mellowed you out. That's all I needed to hear.

"I checked it out the next day and it sounded pretty good. It was a twenty-one-day sleep study that paid about $40. Each night you'd get two sleeping pills, and the next morning before breakfast the doctors would check your vital signs. The pills made me kind of high and then I'd go to sleep. But I was always hungover in the morning and didn't want to go to work."

Fortunately, Butch didn't suffer any ill effects from the study. But neither did it convince him that he could tempt fate and try another clinical trial. His painful experiences at Holmesburg had properly sobered him as to the repercussions of being a human guinea pig.

"I had come to realize," says Butch, "that the tests weren't for me. I only did the sleeping pill test because I was on glue at the time and it sounded like the pills got you high. I didn't do it for the money like the other ones I was on. I learned my lesson and told guys to watch themselves. You could really get fucked up on those tests. I also learned that doctors were full of shit. They couldn't be trusted to have your best interest at heart."

As his release date drew near, Butch stayed out of trouble, did his work in the laundry, and looked forward to the day he'd be able to rejoin his wife and budding family. Laura now had three children, and the third was an issue of some concern. His daughter, Tanya, was born shortly before he went to prison. His second, Edward Jr., was born while he was serving time at Holmesburg, and Butch was pretty much assured he was the father. But the third, Dennis, was born much more recently, and family members quickly changed the subject when asked to describe the baby's physical characteristics. Butch didn't want to think that Laura had been unfaithful, but the conclusion seemed inescapable. He tried not to con-demn her; he knew he hadn't been much of a father. As a drug addict and jailbird, he understood that he was in no position to cast stones.

In mid-1966, after nearly twenty-four months behind bars, Edward "Butch" Anthony had maxed out. A physically and mentally scarred veteran of one of the most violent and bizarre big-city prison systems in the country, Butch had survived the worst two years of his life. Few would have believed the horrors he had endured, but now he was a free man and ready to act like one.

"I was crazy and loose," recalls Anthony of that happy time. "I was ready to party. I was thinking about two things and two things only—a shot of dope and a shot of pussy."

Family members picked him up in front of the House of Correction and drove him back to Laura's house in the heart of North Philadelphia. Although the Village, his native stomping grounds, had witnessed a few changes—none to the community's betterment—Butch paid scant attention, being preoccupied with seeing his wife and children. Laura was as radiant and attractive as ever, but the sight of Dennis, "his" third child, tempered the joyous greeting. The baby had a darker complexion than Butch and the other children, and one could easily discern that he would grow up to be considerably smaller than his siblings.

Fighting the urge to lash out at his wife for her presumed indiscretion and disrupt the happy occasion, Butch left the house, saying he had "people to see," and went around the corner to Vernon's house. A rap on the door and Butch was ushered in with, "Damn, just in time, mother-fucker. We were just fixin' to shoot up." Within two minutes Butch had received his first homecoming shot of heroin.

He then went to his mother's house to greet other family members. It was while there that his pressure shot up—his body was clean, he hadn't had dope in his system in two years—and he collapsed, falling like a statue and banging his head on the floor.

His sister freaked out. "Look at that no-good motherfucker," she screamed. "Doing that shit soon as he gets home."

"You had dope, nigger," said his mother angrily. "You just got home and you're into that shit already. Didn't you learn nothin' in that prison?"

Feeling ill, his head throbbing, angry curses from family members ringing in his ears, Butch staggered back to Laura's place. His long anticipated homecoming was over.

"I Tried My Best"

For many ex-offenders, especially those who have served long sentences in harsh, maximum-security institutions, getting reacclimated to the free world can be a difficult transition. Butch Anthony's nearly two years behind bars were mild by comparison—at least in terms of length—and once on the streets, he hit the ground running. Or in his case, lying down—during his first week of freedom he rarely got out of bed. He and Laura tried to make up for lost time. And getting to know and play with his children brought him more joy than he could have imagined. All five of the Anthonys relished the nonstop hugs and kisses they gave one another.

Butch treated baby Dennis as if he was his own and never brought up the subject of his paternity with Laura. He knew that the issue of her infidelity was highly combustible and might cause a lasting fissure in their relationship. He realized that he was the one who had left them for two years, not the other way around. He hoped to make it up to them.

It was during a family roughhouse session in bed during his first week home that Laura noticed the moist sheets at one end of the bed and asked Butch, "Why are your feet so wet? It's like you just stepped out of the shower."

"I don't know," Butch replied. "It just started this morning. It's like my feet are sweating."

"But you haven't even had any socks or shoes on," said Laura. "What's wrong?"

"It's nothing," said Butch, trying to reassure her. "C'mon back in bed here a little while."

Laura did as Butch requested, but the problem didn't go away—it grew worse. Not only did the areas between his toes remain very wet, but they started to itch. A day later, his hands began to grow moist and itch as well. Soon small red bumps emerged on both

10

his hands and feet. It was as if he had come down with measles. When some of the tiny bumps turned into white pustules, Butch could no longer ignore the obvious—he was suffering a relapse of that first horrible Holmesburg experiment, the skin patch test that made him look like an alien.

"I couldn't believe it," recalls Butch. "It was the same symptoms I had in jail. I was only home a few days and now this was happening to me. I had never had any skin problems. The only time was when I got on that Johnson & Johnson bubble bath test in Holmesburg Prison. Laura saw what was happening and freaked out. She had heard from my sister what I looked like in prison when this shit hit me. And she had seen what I was like on the army study. 'Those damn prison doctors,' she would scream. 'Look what they done to you. Why'd you let them do that to you? They could have killed you in there.' She started to worry that if I didn't go to the hospital right away, these bumps might soon cover my whole body and infect the kids. She was so upset she even told me not to touch the kids.

"I didn't know what to do. I knew I should see a doctor or go to a hospital, but I didn't trust any doctors at that point. And even if I did, I didn't have the money. I had just got home. I applied for my medical assistance card from the welfare office, but it hadn't come in the mail yet.

"Laura kept on tellin' me to see a doctor, but all I felt comfortable doin' was running hot water on my hands and feet to stop the itching. I also put toilet paper between my toes to soak up the sweat and got some different skin creams and lotions from my mother. Nothing worked, but at least the rash didn't progress up my arms and legs. I don't know what I would have done if it started to cover my body like it did in jail. Laura would yell at me every time I went to pick up one of the babies. She was afraid they'd catch it.

"My mom wasn't any more supportive. 'You're a damn fool, Butch,' she would say. 'You gotta stop being a seeker of sensations in life.' She was blaming everything that happened to me as somehow connected to my using drugs. My sister just said, 'Butch, you got no brains. What was you thinking about to let those damn doctors put stuff on you?' With my wife and family screaming at me, I finally promised I'd go to PGH [Philadelphia General Hospital] when the medical card arrived."

Butch did as he had promised and went to the city hospital as soon as the medical card arrived in the mail. A doctor examined him and asked a series of questions, but Butch was reluctant to divulge the fact that this was his second round with this malady. He especially didn't want to mention where he had first contracted it.

"I didn't want everyone knowing my business," says Butch. "When people know you just got out of prison, they treat you different. Besides, I was embarrassed about being on the tests. My family couldn't believe I let myself become a human guinea pig. They were furious. They said it showed how dumb I was, to let people experiment on me."

The PGH physician who examined Butch wasn't quite sure himself what would have precipitated such a dermatological eruption, but he thought the great amount of moisture collecting between his fingers and toes signified some type of weeping eczema. He bathed Butch's hands and feet in a solution and then applied a potent lotion to both extremities. Butch was given a tube of the white cream and told to apply it to the affected areas several times a day. Laura made sure Butch followed the doctor's instructions, and as the days went by the itching began to subside and the tiny red bumps and pustules gradually disappeared. Butch and his family were greatly relieved.

The more he thought about it, though, the more he considered the lotion the PGH doctor had given him a miracle drug, and the angrier he grew thinking about how long he had suffered in Holmesburg. This cream, he thought to himself, had cured him in a fraction of the time he was made to suffer in prison. But inmates weren't given such medication; they were made to suffer.

As Butch's luck would have it, as soon as he overcame one physical malady he came down with another—his hemorrhoid problem recurred. The doctor at Holmesburg had warned him that the surgery might not be a permanent remedy, but he talked himself into believing that, with all he had endured, the problem surely wouldn't return. He was wrong. In fact, the new hemorrhoids were almost as bad as before. Even with all the itching and discomfort, however, he was able to function without alarming those he came in contact with. There was no way of hiding the skin disease, but hemorrhoids were a private matter.

"I just decided I was gonna have to live with it," he says. "I carried Preparation H around with me, and every time I took a shit and the hemorrhoids popped out I just pushed them back in with the cream. After what I went through with those prison doctors, I just decided I ain't lettin' no doctor touch this asshole again."

Now that he was on the way to regaining his health, and with four mouths to feed in addition to his own, he began to feel the pressure to earn some

113

money and start supporting the family. A brother-in-law came through with a decent-paying job for him at Penn Packing, a slaughterhouse at Aramingo and Butler streets in the Kensington section of the city. Butch was assigned an assembly line job, counting and weighing the hogs after their entrails had been taken out. The job paid well and he was contributing to his family's upkeep, but an insidious vice was gradually creeping back into his life—his long and unforgiving addiction to drugs. His normally sound work ethic began to suffer; he'd lose count of the hogs on the conveyor belt, occasionally appear in a drug-induced stupor, and sometimes not show up for work. After two and a half months, he was fired.

In fact, from his first day home, Butch had been shooting up. Friends in the Village normally not known for their generosity were pleased to welcome him home and quick to share their stash of drugs. They'd hang out and talk about how the neighborhood had changed, who was making it and who wasn't, and the increasing number of deaths due to gang violence. Butch, in turn, would give them news of local guys he had seen in jail. Occasionally the discussion would shift to conditions in Holmesburg and Butch's participation in medical experiments. Some had already heard about the research experiments, while others were amazed and said they wouldn't be caught dead letting doctors experiment on them like lab animals. Butch knew the truth: they'd all do it. Desperate people do desperate things.

Within days his friends' generosity had ended, but his habit had not. The job at the meatpacking company paid for his daily shot, but his firing presented a new challenge. Frantic and in need of money, Butch sought out other jobs, but when this proved unsuccessful he resorted to boosting again. Friends encouraged him to join their crews; they were making good scores doing walk-ins and sticking up convenience stores. But Butch wasn't out to hurt anybody. The thought of carrying a gun gave him a chill. He just wanted some money for his habit. He was content ripping off a few resalable items from various commercial establishments. Clothing and appliance stores, as well as supermarkets, were all good to go. He was back in the hustle.

Laura was furious. She hadn't waited two years and struggled raising three children by herself while Butch was in prison for her husband to return to drugs and a life of crime. "How do you think we're gonna live like this?" she would scream at him. "That junk is destroying you and wrecking this family. Oh no, this time it's gonna be different. You're gonna work and support the family. And no fuckin' drugs, you hear?"

Laura was adamant, but Butch was now shooting two, sometimes three bags a day. Neither logic nor threats had an impact. Even his family's welfare had taken a backseat to his need for drugs. An excursion to Harlem with friends to cop some heroin resulted in a three-week stay. It exemplified his abandonment of both reason and responsibility. He had walked out on his employer and his family without a dime's worth of notice.

"I was out of control," says Butch. "When you're on drugs, you can even become an enemy to your loved ones. I just took up and left with Rico and a couple other guys for New York. We got fixed up and just decided to stay. We were so strung out on shit we ended up sleeping in one of those Harlem shooting galleries. The superintendent of an apartment house sold us the dope and said we could crash in the basement of one of his units. It was a real nasty flophouse, with five or six guys sleeping on beds made out of car seats and old, stain-covered mattresses. There were tables filled with shooting paraphernalia: bottle caps for cooking dope, bottles of water, matches, neckties, shoestrings, and ladies' stockings laying all over the place.

"We ended up sleeping in a coal bin in the cellar—a coal bin with a dead body in it. When I first saw this dead guy lying there, I said to myself, what the hell is this? What the fuck did I walk into? I was like Amos and Andy. My eyes popped out of my head. They said the person was dead only a day or two, but they hadn't had time to get rid of the body yet. We slept with this dead person next to us for a couple days. It gave me the creeps, but we were fucked up on drugs and didn't have anyplace else to go."

During those three weeks, Butch and his friends survived by getting painting jobs during the day and doing some boosting on the side. It was far from a glamorous holiday in the Big Apple. "We were all miserable," says Butch. "Just living day to day on the streets of Harlem. You can't believe how bad you feel when you're a junkie. You're always worrying about people catching you and going to prison. And when you're gonna get your next shot. Living like that ain't nothing to get excited about. It's terrible."

After three weeks Butch and his friends decided they had had enough of New York and would go back home to Philly. On his return, Laura was defiant. "I'm not gonna be in this dump much longer," she told him. "You sit around noddin' off when you're supposed to be watching the babies and go off wherever and whenever you want to. And you don't bring no money home for us to live on. You're not gonna be anything but a bum your whole life."

In fact, Laura had started seeing someone else, a cop. She loved Butch, but he was killing himself and his family. She and her babies needed a change.

Butch doesn't dispute the magnitude of his fall. "I was the devil incarnate," he says. "Even when she gave me things to pawn or sell so we'd have some money, I'd use it for drugs. One time she gave me a camcorder to sell and I gave it up for two bags. That shit had me out of control. I had become an enemy to my own family. I didn't know how to stop."

Butch moved back home with his mother. She nagged him mercilessly to get a job, stop doing drugs, and get his life together, but his sister told her to quit wasting her time. Butch was retarded, she'd say, and never going to amount to anything. He continued to boost and shoot dope, and within a short time his unhealthy and illegal lifestyle came to its natural endpoint—Butch was arrested in a Kensington clothing store for shoplifting. Sentenced to a year in jail, he was sent back in Holmesburg Prison.

"I knew everybody in there," says Butch of his second swing through Philadelphia's toughest lockup. "Guys would be welcoming me back, giving me the high fives, and asking if I needed anything. I put on a smile and made pretend I was going with the flow, my being back was no big deal. But I was really ashamed. I couldn't believe I was right back in there again. I may have been joking with the guys and talkin' shit, but I was feelin' uptight, nervous. The Burg was a dangerous place. There was all that coldness and craziness that went on there. I always felt the tension and feared getting hurt. Man, I just couldn't believe I was in there again."

Butch was thrown in a cell with another inmate and given a job in the knit shop. He worked on a weaving machine eight hours a day making bed sheets and inmate uniforms. He earned all of twenty-five cents a day. His meager income was augmented by occasional $10 money orders from his family, but his commissary purchases were still rather paltry. Others on the block suggested he join them on the research studies that were still a vital component of the jail and the main way for inmates to earn money, but Butch had had it with the tests. He had seen enough medical experiments to last a lifetime.

"Oh no," Butch recalls of that second Holmesburg incarceration, "I wasn't going back to those tests. I was finished with that shit. They ruined me the first time. I wasn't going to give them a second crack at me."

If he needed further disincentive it was readily available—both his skin rash and hemorrhoid problems returned only weeks after his arrival. Recurring trips to the prison hospital for salves, ointments, and medical elixirs did little good—jail medications were clearly inferior to what he had received on the street. Complaining and telling the prison doctors what he had been given by PGH doctors for his skin problem were useless. He was a prisoner and would once again have to become accustomed to prison medicine.

"I thought my body would heal," Butch recalls, "but it didn't. I realized I'd be stuck with this shit the rest of my life." .

Butch didn't trumpet his horrendous experiences with the Penn research program throughout the jail; he wasn't a proselytizer. But when bullshit sessions among inmates took place and he was questioned about his reluctance to take part in the studies, he told the truth. "I don't fuck with them no more," he would say, and then go on to recite a few of his experiences. As jaws dropped and listeners became bug-eyed, some inmates refused to believe him and said he was making up stories to alarm them, but others who had been around for a while said the stories were true. They had seen for themselves how Butch's skin eruptions made him look like a hideous monster, and how the army study had turned him into a zombie they called "Outer Limits."

Reactions were always the same. Some men shook their heads in amazement and immediately swore off the tests, while others walked off and hoped Butch's experience was an aberration. The men needed the money and didn't want to hear of experiments gone bad and maimed test subjects. To maintain such optimism, however, meant ignoring the obvious. As Butch says, "so many dudes were getting messed up on the tests, you couldn't help but notice."

A veteran of the institution by now, Butch settled in with a certain crew of guys he felt comfortable with and tried to stay clear of the mayhem and violence that pervaded the jail. "It was the same old crazy shit," he says of his second Holmesburg stint. "Guys were getting stabbed, fights over homos were routine, and card games could always end up in bloodshed. I tried to block it all out and keep to myself whenever I could."

Once again, a key tension reducer, and one of his few social outlets, was music. Butch became friendly with another inmate on the block called Dr. John, who was a whiz with musical instruments, particularly string instruments. He could turn a mop handle, a few feet of string, and a couple nails into an upright bass guitar. At first Butch went to Dr. John's cell to listen to him strum tunes on one of his guitars, but he eventually began accompanying him using two upturned mop buckets. Little by little, other musicians on the block would join the jam sessions, and the four or five imprisoned music makers would really start to pound out the tunes. "Guys would be lining the cell block corridor listening to us," recalls Butch of the impromptu sessions. "Man, we'd really be cookin', and guys couldn't get enough of us. We must have played every day and always had an audience. It really helped relieve the stress."

As the weeks and months slowly passed, Butch had lots of time to think about his life, his family, and how badly he had messed up. He recognized and regretted his mistakes and hoped to make things right, but those sincere moments of remorse were offset by fantasies of getting high again. Butch was a hard-core addict who lusted after his next fix.

"The entire time I was in the Burg," Butch frankly admits, "I couldn't wait till I got out and was able to use drugs again. All I thought about was shooting up again. I had developed a drug mentality. It had become a way of life for me. It was like a religion."

After serving his one-year minimum, Butch was released in September 1968 and got his chance to realize his fantasy. He went back to his mother's house on 27th Street and before the day was done got the shot he had been dreaming of for twelve months. For the next year, Butch's life would be one extended hustle. Boosting food from supermarkets and clothing from department stores, along with the occasional legitimate job, usually lasting no longer than a week or two, provided his income. Stealing from family members could always augment that. In fact, Butch was booted out of his mother's house for doing just that.

His brother Wilbert had a well-paying job and the personal accoutrements that steady employment provides. For Butch, however, his brother's attractive shirts, slacks, and jewelry were a tempting source of money for drugs. Initially he would sneak into his brother's room and swipe a new Ban-Lon shirt or two, but gradually he threw all caution aside and started pilfering his brother's jewelry and money. When he overheard his brother angrily discussing the situation with his mother, Butch tried to make amends—he purchased a new shirt for his brother and placed it on Wilbert's bed. But the well-intentioned gesture was too late; the Anthony family had had enough of its youngest and most troubled member.

Will, a dozen years older and considerably bigger physically, confronted Butch and laid down the law. "This world," he said, "won't be big enough for both of us if you take any of my shit again."

Butch took the threat seriously; his brother would kill him if he were caught stealing any more of his possessions. That possibility, however, became all the more remote when his mother followed up his brother's threat by throwing him out of the house. Mrs. Anthony, the devout Baptist and longtime church activist, was fed up with Butch, fed up with his passion for drugs, his repeated incarcerations, and his lack of support for his wife and kids. His lack of ambition or any sense of personal responsibility infuriated her. She hadn't raised her children to be drug addicts and criminals. It broke her heart, but Butch was a lost soul who was only doing damage to himself and those close to him. He had to be cut loose.

As he exited the house with his few belongings, his mother blistered him with criticisms and told him, "And you stay the hell away from Laura and the kids. Every time you come home that little Tanya has her heart broken. She sees her father, gets attached to you, and then you're gone. You stay away from them, you hear? You've caused enough trouble."

Butch didn't even bother to protest. He knew he had screwed up. He was all too familiar with the thefts, the deceit, and the abandonment of his wife and kids. His recent deception with money Laura had given him to purchase shoes for the kids was a stinging reminder of just how far he had fallen. Instead of getting the kids shoes, he had spent the money on heroin. "I tried my best," Butch told himself, all the while knowing that money for his kids had gone into his vein.

Butch spent the next six months hustling on the streets. He rented a room from a friend for $30 a month, and when he wasn't watching TV he looked for ways to earn money for drugs. It was during this period that Butch began selling drugs for Cadillac Slim, a local drug dealer. Always decked out in sharp clothes and a fashionable hat, and cruising around town in his canary-yellow Eldorado, Cadillac Slim was a conspicuous neighborhood symbol of the rewards of dealing drugs. Butch, however, wasn't interested in designer clothes or fancy automobiles—he wanted the dope. So much so, in fact, that it nearly cost him his life.

Cadillac Slim gave Butch three bundles (twenty-five bags to the bundle) of heroin to sell. Though he made a genuine effort to market the product, his habit got the better of him, and he found himself using more than he sold. When Slim showed up to collect the proceeds, Butch turned over half a bundle, no money, and an apology. Cadillac Slim was livid and threatened to kill Butch on the spot. If Slim hadn't been a close relative

119

who lived around the corner from the Anthony household, Butch would have been discovered on a trash-strewn lot somewhere with a bullet hole in his head.

"The whole thing was humiliating," says Butch of his drug addiction and decision to work with big-time dope dealers. "I had become a masochist. All I thought about was drugs. I couldn't even do a decent job of selling the stuff. I just wanted to use it. I was an addict. I had a disease."

Strangely, the drug-selling fiasco never made it through the Village pipeline. Softheartedness not being a character trait of distinction in the hood, Cadillac Slim didn't want it known that he had been taken without penalizing the perpetrator, so Butch escaped with his life. That bit of luck, however, only contributed to another near catastrophe. With his street reputation seemingly bolstered by his association with Cadillac Slim, Butch was hired by another drug firm, the Warner brothers, to sell dope out of their well-fortified house. Butch was unnerved by the dangerous assignment and by the strange, shady characters always knocking on the door looking to score some heroin. Were they genuine addicts looking to cop, he wondered, or were they stick-up artists looking to make a big score? Or could they be undercover narcotics agents? Nervously sitting by the front door mulling over his precarious situation and eyeballing the bags and bundles of dope strewn before him eventually pushed him over the edge. After three weeks, the danger and temptation caused Butch a minor emotional meltdown.

At first he just tinkered with the contents of some of the bags, teasing out minute portions and then filling a bag or two for himself. As time went on he became bolder and began to rob customers by actually stealing bags from wrapped bundles. He knew the consequences if he was caught; Sidney and Elery Warner were menacing figures in the neighborhood. And they also weren't relatives like Cadillac Slim. If he were caught short-changing customers, or ripping off their stash of drugs or cash, he'd be killed.

He never took a cent of their money, but one day, in a panic, Butch walked off with two bundles of heroin. He then proceeded to pick up his welfare check, pack his bags, and purchase a one-way ticket to New York City, severing his ties to Philadelphia. Harlem, however, proved no more hospitable than his hometown. He wandered the streets looking for a place to stay, exhausting his supply of dope in the process, and contemplated how he was going to survive. Things would get progressively worse.

While walking the streets of Harlem, Butch ran into an old friend from Philly, Jim Yellow. Butch said he had just arrived in town and needed a place to hole up. He also needed a shot. Boasting that he had money for both, Butch convinced Yellow, who was also an addict, to take him to a local dealer and then back to his apartment, where they could shoot up. Butch knew that Harlem heroin was cheaper than it was in Philly, but he forgot that it was also more potent. His friend had to caution him.

"I was about to cook my shot," says Butch, "when Yellow grabbed my arm and said, 'What the hell you doing? You wanna OD? You wanna kill yourself?' He said, 'This is New York shit you're shootin' up with. Just take half a shot, 'cause once you put that shit in your arm, you can't pump it out.' I had been using so much in Philly, almost ten bags a day, that I thought I could handle it. I eased off a bit, but not as much as I should have, because soon as I shot that shit up it was like, *boom*. Man, I fell right out."

Fortunately, Butch didn't die from the overdose. He woke up two days later. Dazed and bewildered, he found himself on the floor in a strange, barren room. When he was finally able to move and collect his thoughts, he realized that he had been taken. His money and dope were gone, and some of his clothes were missing. Whoever had dragged him off and plundered his possessions had even taken his chewing gum.

Broke and desperately in need of money, Butch gravitated to an old hustle in a new city—breaking into cars. He had perfected car break-ins as a juvenile, but the economic landscape of Upper Manhattan was very much different from anything he had known back home. The luxury town-houses and high-rise condominiums surrounding Central Park were fertile fields of opportunity for thieves. The Lincolns, Cadillacs, and snazzy foreign cars parked on the tree-lined streets were an inviting target. Each day he'd travel to a tony section off the park armed with a coat hanger and screwdriver. Rarely did he return to Harlem empty-handed.

"Those rich people living off of Fifth Avenue," Butch recalls, "were always leaving shopping bags filled with stuff in their cars. It was nothing to pop a door lock, grab the bags, and haul ass into the park, where there were rarely cops around. I once did a Jaguar on 92nd Street and pulled out five shopping bags filled with leather coats, expensive sweaters, and a couple boxes of shoes and handbags. It must have been over a thousand dollars' worth of stuff, but all I got for it was $100. The fence I was using was a cheap son of a bitch who ran a candy store in Harlem. One coat alone must have been well over $500, but he only gave me $50 for it. I was getting robbed all the time. I was new to the area; I didn't know anyone else. What could I do?"

The stealing went on for months, mostly on the Upper East and West sides, but occasionally there would be forays through train and bus stations throughout the city. Curiously, Butch ran into a fair number of Philadelphians who were also on the hustle in New York City. "They were dope fiends on the run," says Butch of the contingent of hometown hustlers. "There was Little Dusty from 21st and Norris, George Holder from Camac and Diamond, Mama Too Tight from Ridge Avenue, Seesaw from 17th and Susquehanna, and a bunch of others. New York was the place to go if you were a serious drug addict."

Gradually, the fact that he was "putting his life in jeopardy every day" started to get to Butch. Exhausted, and with more than a tinge of guilt and regret, he wondered if he could stop stealing and make a go of it legitimately. With nothing to lose, he went to a local welfare office. He concocted a sob story, using the name of a distant relative who lived in the Bronx. To his amazement, another welfare officer overheard his story and brought him into her office, reminisced about her years in Philadelphia, and immediately filled out the necessary paperwork. She also wrote him an emergency check for $200.

"She was originally from Philadelphia," says Butch, "and seemed to be interested in helping out somebody in need from her hometown. I couldn't believe she wrote me a check on the spot. Hell, it was twice as much as I ever got from any welfare office in Philly."

Butch took the unexpected good fortune as a sign that he should change his ways and go straight. He got a decent room in an old, run-down hotel called the Kent for $30 a week and immediately sought a legitimate job. Within hours he was hired to deliver orders at Bruce's Restaurant. Hardworking and dependable, Butch was soon stocking shelves and occasionally working as a counter man. The tips alone brought in enough money that he didn't even have to cash his welfare checks, and he periodically took on additional jobs such as silk-screening. Butch was doing much better, but he was still addicted to heroin.

"Yeah, I was doing better and had cut out a lot of that crazy stuff I was doing," he says, "but I was still shooting fifteen $2 bags a day. I was a dope fiend. Everything was based on the next day's fix."

"I Was in Some Deep Shit Now"

Though his intentions were good, Butch's half-hearted, incremental attempts to clean up his act were destined to fail—he just wasn't prepared psychologically or ready spiritually to get clean, break with his criminal past, and establish a healthy, crime-free life for himself. Moreover, things seemed to happen to Butch that happened to few others. He always seemed to be in the wrong place at the wrong time, when the wrong thing was happening. Even when he had no inclination or intention to break the law, a criminal act seemed to find him.

His introduction to the New York City criminal justice system is a perfect example. "We were walking down the street," says Butch matter-of-factly of the event that would culminate in his first bust in the Big Apple. "I was with George Olden, another old junkie from Philly who was up in Harlem to cop drugs. We had just turned onto Broadway when we seen the sidewalk littered with furniture. There were boxes and sofas and chairs and televisions all over the place, you could just about walk through without bumping into something. A furniture store was getting a delivery of goods, and the sidewalk and half the street was cluttered with stuff. Then we saw these two Puerto Rican guys come out of the store, grab a large box holding a television, and carry it into the store. I ain't paying any particular attention to any of this, when George looks over at me and says, 'We can swing some of this.'

"'What?'

"'You heard me,' he says. 'If we hurry, we can swing some of this stuff.'

"'Man, are you crazy?'

"'C'mon, Butch,' says George. 'The stuff is just sittin' out here.'

"'Forget it, man,' I tell him, 'you think we're gonna run off with a chaise lounge or television?'"

Just then George Olden gave Butch a look like he didn't know what he was talking about and then took hold of one end of a large cardboard box containing an Admiral Hi-Fi TV set. He started dragging it while yelling at Butch to grab the other end. Initially stunned by the old man's audacity on a busy public street, Butch was both speechless and seemingly unable to move.

"C'mon nigger," yelled George, "I can't move this heavy motherfucker by myself. Grab the other end."

With Olden urging him on, Butch quickly scanned the store entrance for any workers and grabbed the other end of the box. His adrenalin pumping, Butch was up and running, or at least moving as fast as he could with a bulky, hundred-pound item that is further weighed down by a sixty-year-old drug addict whose spirit is decidedly more willing than his body.

"We don't get a half-block," says Butch, "when I see them tear ass out of the store after us. These Puerto Rican boys and these other white guys who must have been the store's owners are running down the street after us and yelling at us to stop. I'm screaming at George to hurry and pick up his end, but he's already winded, and the box is getting closer and closer to the ground. He's about to drop it any second and I'm yelling at him, 'They're coming, c'mon, c'mon,' but this old nigger that started this shit is dead on his feet. He would have fallen on his ass if it wasn't for the Puerto Ricans grabbing him. I dropped the other end of the box and grabbed George's other arm and we're both pulling him, me one way and the Ricans the other. Old skinny George must've looked like a dried stick that was being pulled by two thin twigs. Every time they tried to grab me, I raised my fist and they backed off, but they wouldn't let go of George's arm."

With some additional Puerto Rican employees who had joined the chase screaming in Spanish and the storeowners about to pounce on Butch, he was forced to abandon the old man and try to save himself. He started running as fast as his legs could carry him. Track meets of this nature down Harlem's Amsterdam Avenue weren't all that unusual, but this was Butch Anthony's maiden sprint as the prey in New York City, and he felt like he was running for his life.

"Man, I broke from ol' George when I saw what was coming," says Butch of the frightening episode. "I was humping down Amsterdam Avenue like a slave outta Georgia, but those Puerto Rican boys were right on me. I turned into an apartment building near a construction site and thought about climbing to the roof, 'cause that was a favorite trick in Harlem when folks

124

Sentenced To Science

were on your tail, but I figured I'd outsmart them by hiding behind the first-floor staircase and watch them make the climb for nothing.

"But my luck that day was all bad. While three ran up the stairs, two stayed behind on the first-floor landing. I could hear them yapping in Spanish and started to get the feeling they knew I was right around the corner from them. Man, I thought to myself, I better make a break for it before the others come back down and I got no chance at all.

"I pulled out my screwdriver that I carried to break into cars, stepped into the hallway and said to them, 'Listen muthafuckers. If you don't get out of my muthafuckin' way I'm gonna stab your ass.' Their eyes got big as turkey pots. As I moved to the front door, one of them swung a shovel that he had picked up on the street outside and tried to take my head off with it. I got my arm up just in time and the shaft of the shovel broke. It woulda hurt like hell, but the adrenalin was running, and I just pushed them out of the way and ran through the doorway like a crazy man and out on to the street.

"I was running like an Olympic sprinter, but those dudes wouldn't give up. Cursing and yelling in Spanish as they chased after me, we musta run five blocks, and I didn't know what I was gonna have to do to get away from them. I didn't wanna hurt anybody, but I knew I didn't wanna get hurt myself."

The chase ended when a large green van suddenly pulled in front of Butch on a Harlem side street and five members of New York City's elite police SWAT team jumped out of the vehicle with guns drawn. Butch was quickly subdued, handcuffed, and taken to the back of the van. When the police opened the doors to the van he was surprised to see George Olden lying on the floor next to the Hi-Fi box.

"Is this your father?" asked one of the officers.

"Hell no," Butch replied. "I ain't ever seen that muthafucker before."

Butch's feeble attempt at deception was as effective as his thievery. He was taken to the Tombs in Lower Manhattan, made to sit in a basement bullpen overnight, and taken before a magistrate the next morning who set a trial date. Butch had heard stories about the Tombs and braced himself for some uncomfortable hours. Flashbacks to his early days at Holmesburg came to mind, forcing him to be cognizant of how he should carry himself, what he should be on the lookout for, and how he should respond if threatened. Butch was a new fish in America's largest urban jail; he knew he had to be prepared for anything.

"I Was in Some Deep Shit Now"

To his surprise, he adapted rather well. Not that the Tombs, where he spent a month, and Rikers Island, where he did another three months, were a walk in the park. Both were tough, unforgiving big-city jails holding the usual array of social miscreants, from down-and-out vagrants to outright killers and sociopaths. Inmates were brutalized by other inmates, correctional officers were far from lenient, progressive-minded social workers, and conditions were Spartan at best. But Butch was no novice— his prison demeanor had already been forged in one of the toughest jails on the East Coast.

"It was the same sort of craziness at Rikers that I had seen at Holmesburg," says Butch. "Their prisons weren't nearly as old as the Burg, but the inmates were the same, and the guards were tough and would fuck you up in a second. There were always fights among the inmates, especially over who would get to use the TV and what they were going to watch. But with all the stuff going on, they left me alone. Guys in New York thought everyone in Philly could fight. Guys who went to Philly and did time came back to New York and found they had made a rep for themselves. They considered the whole damn town a school for gladiators and usually left anybody from Philly alone. That was just fine with me. I just wanted to do my time and get out."

Another pleasant surprise was the absence of any prison testing; there was no scientific research going on. The jails in Philly were practically enveloped by research protocols, but New York had none. Butch pondered the difference for some time. Why were medical experiments pervasive in one urban prison system and nonexistent in another, just ninety miles away? Rikers Island was loaded with prisons holding many more inmates than were being held captive in Philly. And the inmates were all desperate to earn some money. Why wouldn't they be experimenting on people here? Butch finally concluded that it could only be due to one thing. "Philly had the University of Pennsylvania and New York didn't."

Butch was released after four months, but he had had no epiphany during his incarceration. He was still a drug addict and his life was still a hustle. He needed a shot of heroin, some money, and a place to stay. With any luck, he might be able to pick up another emergency check from the welfare office and talk his way into another room at the fleabag Harlem hotel where he'd been staying before he fell. To his amazement, he discovered that the hotel had kept his room intact—the reward for always paying his rent on time and being a good tenant. But management now demanded the rent money that was owed.

While looking for ways to make some quick money, Butch learned that George Olden—who had gotten out of prison a month earlier—was in bad shape and hospitalized in Harlem Hospital. He wanted to visit George, but Butch was now perpetually nervous around doctors and had developed a serious fear of hospitals. Forcing himself to overcome his fears, Butch saw George, but the old man was failing badly. Diabetes, combined with extensive use of street drugs, had caused several organs to fail. Butch tried to cheer the old man up, but his efforts were futile. Olden died just two days after the visit.

It was while he was trying to negotiate an emergency check from the welfare office that he ran into another Rikers graduate. The former inmate had just picked up his welfare check and expressed his intention to cop some drugs, but he lacked one thing—a place to stay; he was homeless. A good ten to fifteen years older than Butch, "the guy was stocky, dark-skinned, with strong African features." He had a gift for gab and a friendly, knowledgeable demeanor, and Butch figured there were worse characters to hang out with. The two men discussed their assets and needs and quickly decided to share their respective resources—Butch would get the dope he desired and his newfound friend would get a temporary roof over his head. The spur-of-the-moment relationship would culminate in one of the most unusual and harrowing events in Butch Anthony's life.

127

"The guy was a cocaine freak," says Butch. "I personally never liked the stuff and never used it. I had tried it a couple times and always got sick from it. I really wanted some heroin, but I let this guy run the show. He knew his way around and seemed to know everyone. We went to see some people he knew, copped some coke, and shot up back at my place. Now I'm all messed up. The coke did nothing but make me sick, as usual. He said, 'Let's go make some money,' so I followed him down to Grand Central Station, where we found a car loaded with shopping bags and a suitcase. There were some nice cashmere sweaters and coats with fur collars inside, certainly enough to score another shot or two.

"The guy then takes me over to a cab company he once worked for up around 125th near Amsterdam, and he's making small talk with some of the drivers and the dispatcher. We then go to the back of the lot and he tells me to get in one of the taxicabs. Before I know it, this guy is driving us off the lot and out into traffic. He just stole one of the cars. I'm tellin' you, this guy was really something.

"We're driving around Manhattan like we own it. Fifth Avenue and the Metropolitan Museum of Art, all the fancy shops on Madison Avenue, around Central Park and the ritzy high-rise apartments, the Plaza, Carlyle, and Waldorf-Astoria hotels, he really knew the town. He's showing me places I never been but only heard about, and he keeps talking about how we're gonna make some money. He then drives over to this ice cream warehouse where they load trucks to distribute ice cream around the city, and he pulls behind this one truck. He tells me to get out, and in just a few minutes we had popped the door and filled the taxi with twenty to thirty boxes of ice cream. The shit was frozen solid. There were Popsicles, Creamsicles, Fudgsicles, Dixie cups, bottles of milk and orange juice. Man, we had it all. The cab's backseat and trunk was packed with all kinds of stuff, and I'm laughin' and wondering what the hell we're gonna do with it all.

"He then drives around Harlem and parks by a high-rise apartment complex near 127th and Lennox. He finds one of those old supermarket carts, we load it up with the stuff we just stole and go up to the top floor of the apartment building. We went door to door and floor by floor from the fourteenth floor to the bottom of the building, selling ice cream, milk, and orange juice at steep discounts. Must have made three trips back to the car to reload. A half-gallon of milk for half the price the stores charged, boxes of Fudgsicles for a fraction of what anybody would be really paying for them. Sometimes little raggedy-assed kids would open the door and we'd ask if their mama was home 'cause we were sellin' stuff cheap. My friend would just go knocking at the next apartment if no adults with money were home, but I'd end up givin' the kids a Popsicle or something. I felt like Santa Claus. My friend would yell at me for givin' the profits away, but I figured we didn't pay for it, and some of these kids looked in worse shape than me. Anyway, by the time we got back to the ground floor, our fists were full of cash. We had made a couple hundred bucks and could really party now."

The two street hustlers went back to Butch's shabby hotel room at 115th Street and 8th Avenue, but not before buying a few necessities—a $20 bag of coke for his friend and two bags of dope for Butch. The festivities took a surprising turn when they arrived back at his hotel, where they were met by four of Butch's friends from Philly—Barge, Fats Cradle, Clayvon, and Geech. They had just come up to Harlem, copped some dope themselves, and now wanted a safe place to shoot up. All were in a good mood and eager for the party to get started. Everyone shot up, heroin for Butch and the Philly contingent, coke for his Rikers pal. The only sour note sounded when Clayvon asked if she could share some of the coke. She was rudely rebuffed, which caused a few tense moments. Nearly six feet tall and athletically built, Clayvon came from a family of North Philly toughs who didn't take insults lightly.

"Okay, motherfucker," said Clayvon. "If that's the way you want to be, you stingy son of a bitch."

Butch and his Philly friends thought Clayvon was going to take a swing at the guy. Men didn't intimidate her. The mix of drugs and ill will only exacerbated the tension in the room.

Butch began nodding, a typical result of shooting dope, and grew irritated that his Rikers friend was playing the music too loud and dancing around the room like Bojangles Robinson. The coke had this brother up and feeling no pain, while his compatriots on heroin were having difficulty keeping their heads up and their eyes open. Periodically Butch managed to lift his head and spy his light-footed guest dancing around as if he hadn't a care in the world. But then he'd nod off again.

A sudden noise, however, caught Butch's attention, and he half-noticed his new friend now standing stiff as a board with a weird grimace on his face, as he firmly grasped a hot plate in one hand and, in the other, a gas line leading to a small stove in a corner of the room. The man then began shaking violently, his eyes growing large as saucers, the metal hot plate crumpling in his hand as if crushed by a large vice. Butch and the others weren't sure what was happening, but once the man keeled over and hit the floor with a loud thud, it didn't take a forensic pathologist to determine that he had suffered a drug-induced seizure. Flat on his back and shaking violently, he vibrated across the room as if possessed by a supernatural force, causing the others to scatter and cry out, "Watch out," "Get out of the way," "He's OD-ing."

Butch yelled out, "Oh my God. What's happening?" as he fought to throw off the effects of the heroin that was now coursing through his body.

"Man, he's shakin' like a motherfucker," said Fats Cradle as he jumped out of the way.

"Fuck that nigger," Clayvon shouted, still angry over the cocaine snub. "I hope the son of a bitch drops dead."

As Butch bent over his fallen friend to try and provide the man some assistance, Geech said, "Butch, you can't do nothin' for that nigger. He's had it. He's gone."

"I Was in Some Deep Shit Now"

129

"No he's not. He's still alive," Butch insisted, straddling the man, slapping his face, and performing chest compressions in an attempt to revive him. "Help me. Help me get him up."

"Forget it," said Geech. "You can throw that motherfucker out in the trash."

Panic-stricken and still fighting the effects of the dope, Butch was beside himself. "I didn't want to see this muthafucker die on me," he recalls. "I didn't know what to do for him, and the others just stood around watching. I couldn't believe this motherfucker that had just showed me around Manhattan, and I had just done all this stuff with, was dropping dead on me. He was still breathin' and I thought he still had a chance, but then this nigger looked up at me like he had just seen the sun come up. And that was it. He was gone.

"Lord have mercy, I thought to myself. I'm in some deep shit now. I'm gonna go to prison for manslaughter. I'm walking around the room, cursing my lousy luck, and wondering what I'm gonna do with this here dead nigger lying on the floor. The others were no damn help at all.

"Clayvon said, 'Served that nigger right,' and Geech kept on tellin' me to throw him out in the trash. Barge said, 'If you don't get rid of that nigger quick, they're gonna take your black ass to jail.'

"I didn't know what to do.

"Clayvon and Geech started going through the guy's pockets. They took all the money we had just made selling that damn ice cream and then started taking the guy's clothes off. I asked him what the hell did he think he was doing, and Geech said the guy was better dressed than he was, so he was gonna take 'em. I couldn't believe it. He totally strips this guy naked and starts getting in this dead guy's clothes. I began yelling at them that instead of ripping this guy off they should be helping me think of ways to get rid of this guy and to put some clothes on him. We started arguing with each other, and they said, 'Fuck you—take care of this dead nigger yourself,' and they all started walking out on me.

"I said, 'You ain't gonna leave this nigger here dead and naked,' but they did. I didn't know what the fuck to do. All I knew was that I was in some deep shit now. Man, as the hours went by, you can't imagine how depressed I got. I figured I was going back to prison. And as I walked around the room tryin' to figure out how to get out of this mess, I had visions that the guy was following me. In the meantime, the body is getting hard and starting to swell up. He looked like he was now five hundred pounds.

"Later that night, there's a knock at the door. My heart stopped. I thought it was the cops comin' to get me. But it was Barge. He came back. He said he couldn't leave me with that body in the room. He said we could get rid of it by waiting till everyone was asleep in the building and then taking the body up to the roof, leavin' it there, and calling the police the next day, and tellin' them that there's a body on the roof. I didn't have any better ideas, so I said okay."

Butch and Barge waited till about three in the morning before embarking on their dangerous nocturnal mission. If caught, they'd both be facing some serious prison time. Just wrapping the body in a bed sheet proved taxing, as rigor mortis was well under way and the bloating made an already difficult and loathsome chore that much worse. Butch's third-floor room was only one flight from the roof, but neither man had experience with such a tricky endeavor. Checking the hallway for any signs of life, the cautious duo began to transport their recently departed human cargo.

"I was scared to death," Butch recalls of that chilling ordeal. "I was nervous as all hell as we entered the hallway. I was holding the heaviest part, the guy's chest and shoulders. Barge was in front of me holding the legs and feet. The body was damn heavy, and so stiff it didn't even bend as we started taking him up the steps to the roof. It was like a big, heavy log. I was paranoid and kept on lookin' behind me to see if anyone was coming out of their room, and Barge is whispering loudly to stop lookin' around and keep my mind on what we were doin'. The body was heavy as hell and getting heavier as we went up the stairs. I swear, it seemed like I was carrying this sucker by myself; all the weight seemed to be at my end.

"Then, about halfway up the stairs, that dead muthafucker farted. Man, it was a loud, stinkin' fart that nearly caused me to pass out right on the spot. Barge, who was lookin' the other way, said, 'Stop that shit.'

"I told him, 'That wasn't me. That was this dead nigger we're carryin'. This guy's body must have been so filled with gases that moving him up the stairs like we were doin' just caused him to fire the mother of all farts. It hit me square in the face and I nearly lost my balance and staggered against the wall. The smell was terrible. I nearly fainted. Barge started to yell at me to keep moving, we were almost at the top, but I was about to pass out. The odor was incredible. I started to gag and thought I was going to vomit.

"'C'mon, don't stop,' says Barge, 'we're almost there.' I'm strugglin' to hold on to this dude, but I couldn't help myself. I started to throw up. It

131

was only light at first, but by the time we got up on the roof my guts were really pouring out of me. Between the heroin, the guy dying on me, and the smell of that awful goddamn fart, it was amazing I didn't pass out myself.

"Fortunately, it was real cold that night, and snowing, and the fresh air sort of revived me. When I was through vomiting and had got myself together a little, Barge said, 'Let's move the body to the next roof.' We put the body near some cardboard and junk that was scattered up there and Barge then laid a set of works near the guy. We quietly went back to my room and waited. Barge fell asleep, but I was too emotionally strung out to sleep. All I kept thinkin' was, why does all this crazy shit keep happening to me?

"As soon as Barge woke up the next morning, I asked him when we gonna call the cops. Barge said we'd wait and hope somebody else would come across him, but if they didn't, we would have to do it. I was nervous as hell and kept on encouraging Barge to make the call. Late that afternoon, when it was getting dark outside, he went to a phone booth on the street and called the police. He told 'em, 'Hey, there's a dead body on the roof.' We waited and waited, but the police never came. I couldn't believe it.

"Finally, the next morning, the police showed up. They took a look, then went back to their cars and drove off. I couldn't understand why they left this guy out there like that. It was snowing like crazy now. Later that night, many hours later, some different police and city workers showed up and finally removed the body. They put him in a bag and rolled him down the stairs. They didn't bother carryin' him, they just rolled him down three flights of stairs like he was a bag of potatoes. I couldn't believe how they were treatin' him. I did dumb stuff, but I was a functional illiterate and a junkie. These were police officers. They were supposed to do things the right way.

"When I finally saw them lift the body into the back end of a police wagon and take my friend away, I realized I didn't even know the guy's name."

Such a traumatic experience should have been enough to motivate Butch to get off drugs and clean up his life, but it wasn't—he was still enveloped in the web of addiction and bad decisions. With little hope or positive direction in his life and a still-evolving conscience, he seemed destined for more of the same. For a hard-core inner-city addict like Butch Anthony, it would take more than a friend's death to bring a life-altering personal epiphany. There was certainly no shortage of potential stimuli, however.

Just two weeks after the deadly overdose, Butch made a critical mistake while shooting up and developed a severe infection. He was in the process of injecting himself with heroin when he missed his vein and accidentally pumped the potent narcotic into his muscle. There seemed no harm at first, but the wound soon began to abscess, became discolored, and ballooned in size. He knew he was in trouble when home remedies proved inadequate and the pain and swelling increased. Seeking medical attention was an option of last resort, if not completely out of the question. The Holmesburg experience had seared his psyche; doctors were likely to make things worse rather than better.

"Man, I couldn't believe what I had done to myself," says Butch of that painful episode. "My arm blew up to the size of my leg. The pain was terrible, and I had to quit the restaurant on Hudson Street I was working at. I couldn't carry anything, it throbbed all the time, and if anybody accidentally bumped into it I nearly passed out. I kept hoping the pain would subside and it would get better on its own, but it was actually getting worse. I needed to work 'cause I was running out of money and knew I was gonna be thrown out of my hotel room. I knew I should go to a hospital and see a doctor, but I was afraid of them. I was frightened they'd use me as a guinea pig again. They'd see this problem I had and try to do some crazy stuff with me. I didn't want them touching me.

"I kept thinking this way until a friend came over to my place and saw my arm. He was amazed and said I had a bad fuckin' problem and I better get to a doctor before I lose the arm. I knew it was bad, but his reaction really got me worried. I told him how I felt about doctors and some of the shit they did to me in prison. He sympathized but said what I was doing was just making things worse. He said maybe I'd get lucky and find a good doctor that really cared about me and that they weren't all like the ones who were working in Holmesburg Prison.

"He convinced me to go to the emergency unit at Manhattan General. I told the doctor I had fallen on the cement sidewalk while delivering a lunch order, but the doctor was no fool. After asking me a few questions and checking me out, he said, 'Are you sure this wasn't from a puncture wound?' I continued to lie, but the more he examined my arm, the more convinced he became it was a needle puncture that had caused my arm to swell up to the size of an elephant's leg. I think he suspected I was a heroin addict.

"He told me he'd give me some pain medicine and antibiotics for the arm, but only if I let him put me in Manhattan General's detox program. I was in a lot of pain and wanted the medicine. I figured I had no choice, so I said okay and let him admit me into the hospital's drug program.

"It was a twenty-one-day deal, and the first time ever I was on methadone. They were just substituting one form of dope for another, if you ask me. We were noddin' off just like with the real stuff. They put me in a room with two other guys, a homosexual and a Chinese dude who was always crying as he went through withdrawal. We were all pretty fucked up. I know I was jonesin'. My arm gradually got better and started looking like an arm again, but they had to give me chlorohydrate at night so I could sleep. There was a lot of counseling going on. Some of it was one on one and some was group therapy sessions.

"Some dudes really wanted to kick, but I think most guys were in the program just to cut down on their habits. It was costing them too much money. Methadone would let them cold-turkey their way back to a few bags a day rather than ten or twelve they were doing on the street. They didn't want to kick their habit; they just wanted it at a manageable level, something they could afford.

"After the twenty-one days, they kicked me out of there. No sooner had I walked out of the hospital and hit the street than I saw a couple of other guys who had just left the program out on the sidewalk with a bottle of Thunderbird. They were celebrating their escape and lookin' to score their next fix. Guys still in the program could see us from their rooms in the hospital and were callin' out to us to take a nip for them. We toasted them with a couple swigs of wine and then went on our way, but I had nowhere to go. I had lost my hotel room and was out of money. I was in bad shape."

Homeless, poverty-stricken, and increasingly disillusioned with his life in New York, Butch went to a couple of welfare offices looking for assistance, but this time there was none to be had. In fact, his meager circumstances were further aggravated when he temporarily hooked up with another street hustler and his teenage hooker and was scammed out of his last few dollars.

After six months, the Big Apple had turned decidedly sour. Edward "Butch" Anthony had had enough of New York City and the constant struggle to make ends meet. He was now ready to return home to Philadelphia. But how? He had no money or way of getting back. After several unsuccessful attempts to get help at various Travelers Aid societies, he was overheard begging for a ticket home at Manhattan's midtown bus terminal by an elderly African American gentleman. After listening to a lengthy and heartrending account of his screwed-up life—Butch refers to it as a "sob story"—the old man purchased a bus ticket for his distraught, down-and-out acquaintance.

When Butch got off the bus two hours later at the Greyhound terminal in Center City, Philadelphia, he fell to his knees and kissed the ground as if he was a member of the armed forces returning from combat duty in a war-torn land. "I was so glad to be back," recalls Butch, "that I forgot all the things that were waitin' for me."

It wouldn't be long, however, before reality would come back to smack him in the face. An outstanding sheriff's warrant, an embittered parent and resentful spouse, and a rapidly declining, crime-ridden neighborhood awaited his arrival.

"My mom let me have it as soon as I walked in," Butch recalls. "I hadn't bothered to stay in touch all that time I was in New York, and now she really dropped it on me.

"'Your wife has papers for you to sign. She's getting a divorce and I don't blame her one bit. You abandoned her and the babies. You sign 'em and you stay away from her kids. You're no good for them, so you stay the hell away from them or I'll throw you out of my house. I'm tellin' you, you better get a job, stay clear of any drugs and criminals, or you'll be out on your lazy ass. I'm only lettin' you stay here because it's less likely you'll get in trouble this way. But I'm warning you, if I see any drugs . . .'"

Butch got a shot of heroin the next day, caught up on things that had happened while he was away, discovered who was in jail and who was out, and started thinking about making some money. Within days he had nailed down a job as a "spotter" for Black Moochie, a drug dealer in the neighborhood, who paid Butch to "talk up" the quality of Moochie's stash. The nascent business relationship worked for a time, but a conscientious cop and a busted headlight put a stop to the arrangement.

While driving down 29th Street one evening in one of Moochie's beat-up cars, one that lacked a front headlight, among other things, a police cruiser pulled up behind Butch with lights flashing. Knowing that he was wanted for an outstanding warrant and light on identification at the time, Butch panicked, hit the gas, and laid rubber while turning the corner onto Susquehanna Avenue. With little experience behind the wheel, Butch was soon boxed in by the cruiser and forced to stop. As Butch lacked both

135

proper identification and a driver's license, the police officer called in to headquarters and discovered the outstanding warrant.

Back home for only a couple of months, Butch found himself in the Philadelphia Prison System yet again. For the next year he would call the House of Correction home, but this time he would have a new kind of life-altering experience—he would become a convert to Islam.

"My Spiritual Awakening"

Though raised by hardworking, God-fearing parents and encouraged to lead a decent, sober life, Edward "Butch" Anthony was about to close out the 1960s in jail. A shiftless high school dropout and drug addict, Butch had become a habitual offender whose only interest in life was his next shot of heroin. No longer did he feel embarrassment on entering Holmesburg, the House of Correction, or the Detention Center; he had become a hard-core repeat offender. Though his offenses were relatively modest compared to those of the men with whom he shared the cell blocks and dormitories, he had cemented his position as social refuse, a piece of human flotsam floating periodically in and out of the city's burgeoning prison system.

Faced with another year behind bars, Butch decided he'd try and make the best of a bad situation by staying out of trouble, taking advantage of the prison system's few programs, and keeping himself as far away as possible from researchers and their bizarre medical studies. His plan seemed to go awry immediately, however, when he was placed in a cell with a tall, well-built inmate who displayed as stern a face and intimidating a demeanor as he had ever come across in jail. Casting hard looks or "gritting" on other inmates in a show of manly bravado was part of the game, nothing he hadn't been exposed to a thousand times before. But this time was different.

"I thought for sure me and this guy were gonna go at it," says Butch of the grim, humorless inmate. "I had already seen him on the cell block when we were receiving orientation. Most guys were acting like party time. Being in prison was no big deal to them. It was a block of nuts and screwballs, but this one guy was as severe as a heart attack. No smile, no comment, no nothing. He seemed to wanna be separate from everybody. People just tried to stay clear of him. I

12

thought to myself, man, I sure as hell don't wanna lock up with this stern-faced muthafucker. And who do I end up celling with? Just my fuckin' luck. I figured me and this guy are gonna go at it in no time at all.

"I saw he had a few books laying out on his bunk, so I thought I'd try and break the ice and make some conversation. Since they looked like some kind of religious or self-help books, I said, 'You into astrology? Me and a couple of other guys been talkin' about the stars and planets and what our futures look like.'

"Not a word. He turned and looked at me like I just walked out of OBS in a straitjacket. I figured I shouldn't press the issue or we're gonna rumble right here, so I just started unpacking my few things on the bunk, cursing my lousy luck under my breath and wondering how I'm gonna explain to the guards I need a transfer to another cell."

In his late twenties, like Butch, the dour inmate was taller and sported the bushy Afro hairstyle popular at the time. A sturdy build and graceful, athletic movements that could only mean trouble in a physical confrontation complemented his deadly serious demeanor. A few minutes of uncomfortable silence passed, when suddenly two books were tossed onto Butch's bunk and he heard his stern cell mate proclaim, "Astrology is for the weak of mind. If you're serious about the world and your place in it, if you want to know where we've been and where we're headed, this is what you should be reading." Butch was unfamiliar with the books, but his cell mate's first utterance was the beginning of an educational and religious tutorial that would last a lifetime.

"At first," recalls Butch, "I was fascinated by the way he spoke. He sounded like Orson Welles or one of those British actors, with every word out of their mouth sounding like it was coming down from on high. The man had diplomacy and presence. He was one of the most eloquent people I had ever heard. It was English, all right, but it was spoken with such authority and conviction. He was talking about man's fate, the foolish things people believe, injustices taking place throughout the world, and what one has to do to change the course of his life. I'm telling you, the man was mean. He could really spit it out.

"For the next twenty-four hours, we didn't do anything else but talk about the great issues of the day, important events taking place in the world, and man's need for divine guidance and spirituality. We discussed everything from reincarnation and religion to race relations and the problems of the cities. He taught me about Allah and what Islam really was, not the bastardized version of Elijah Muhammad and what his followers were pushing on the cell blocks. He said God created everyone and there was good and bad in every race. He didn't go around calling the white man the devil. He said such notions were a sign of ignorance. The real Islam was about peace and the never-ending quest to achieve it. He said the pen was mightier than the sword, and anything written that called for violence and racial hatred wasn't worth the paper it was written on.

"The man was truly deep. His presence and charisma were overpowering. He was so articulate and impressive. I had never met anyone like him in jail before. He told me his name was Lester Overstreet, but he wanted me and everyone else to call him by his Islamic name, Khalil Abdul Mustafa. He had been up at Rockview [State Prison] for some time and was about to be released. He had run the law clinic up there and was really down with the law. He was a serious jailhouse lawyer and had gotten a lot of guys out of prison. He was probably more knowledgeable about writs and appeals than real lawyers on the street. He showed me one letter from Juanita Kidd Stout, a Court of Common Pleas judge, saying he was helping so many guys in prison it looked like he was practicing law without a license.

139

"But it was really his knowledge of Islam that caught my interest and the subject we spent the most time discussing. It was the beginning of my spiritual awakening. Brother Khalil overwhelmed me with the true Islam, not that crap the Black Muslims had been spreading in the jails. The only thing I and most others knew of Islam is what we heard from Elijah Muhammad and the Black Muslims. Khalil said they were spewing out hatred, dogma, and lies. All of that stuff about Fard Muhammad coming down to earth to instruct Elijah Muhammad how to lead the lost and found black man out of the wilderness of North America into salvation was pure bunk.

"He said Allah was the true God of Islam. Omnipotent and omnipresent, Allah was the creator of the heavens and the universe and everything else. He was the same God that created Adam, the father of the human race, and the one who sent Abraham, Moses, Jesus, and all the prophets with the same message—Islam is the religion of peace, and under Islam all races and peoples are equal.

"Khalil would open some of his books and show me passages to support what he was saying. In fact, he showed me the sixteenth verse of John in the

Bible, where it foretold the coming of the prophet Muhammad, who would lead mankind into the truth of all things. And that's why Muhammad is known as the last prophet and there would be no other after him.

"He told me how the archangel Gabriel enlightened Muhammad as a young man and guided him in becoming a head of state and in the promulgation of laws for his people. According to him, Muhammad was different than all the other prophets in that he was successful during his lifetime. It didn't take centuries for his importance to become evident.

"Man, the whole thing was incredible. Hour after hour we talked about religious concepts, why and what people believed, and how one should live their life. It was really eye-opening. I felt for the first time that I was beginning to understand what it was all about. Brother Khalil taught me so much that first day and night. He explained what made a good Muslim and how one had to make a declaration of faith that was based on the Five Pillars of Islam, which consisted of bearing witness that there was no other God than Allah; praying five times a day; contributing a percentage of your income to the needy; fasting from sunup to sundown one month a year; and making a pilgrimage to Mecca at least once during your lifetime.

"Khalil said if you became a devout Muslim and followed Muhammad's teachings, Allah would forgive you for all your past sins.

"Man, after listening to Khalil rap about all these spiritual things, I thought I was talking to Moses. He gave me lessons every day and every night. He did something to me spiritually. He really opened me up. I was like a sponge. I took in everything he said. I was reborn in that joint. When I was a young kid, my parents worked so hard to follow church teachings and encouraged me to do the same, but the church didn't do anything for me. What I heard in church either frightened me or made no sense. But this experience really changed me. It turned me around.

"Man, it was amazing how many topics we covered. Even in areas outside of Islam, what Khalil said had a profound effect on me. He'd watch me put various creams and lotions on my body and my constant use of Preparation H and said it looked like I was involved in some kind of ritual. When I told him it was all because of the damn prison experiments, he said if I had been a practicing Muslim I would have known what to do. Islam teaches you to safeguard your body and not abuse it. He said I would have instinctively known to say no to the doctors. This country, he said, was based on usury, hypocrisy, and phony institutions. One always had to be vigilant and aware of charlatans looking to cheat and harm us. Paying us chump change for a little piece of our skin was an example of that.

"I gradually bought into the Islamic principles. Some of the hardest for me were the ones dealing with taking care of my body and not introducing any foreign substances into it. A lot of guys on the block were huffing glue, making prison wine, and everybody smoked cigarettes. I tried damn hard to stop drugs and smoking. I nearly had a nervous breakdown trying to kick that stuff, but I forced myself to do it. The experience was so deep.

"As time went on, my interaction with all the other inmates changed. I was more serious, I didn't play around anymore, and the other guys on the block acted accordingly. I got respect for trying to improve myself. The brothers behaved themselves around me. I believe the spirit of God was working through me.

"Even my wife noticed. Laura and I were now divorced, but I started writing her from prison. She couldn't believe what she was reading in those letters, but they must have intrigued her, because she came up to see me. After fifteen or twenty minutes of the visit, she said, 'Wow, you're beautiful. Your mind has really opened up.'"

There can be no doubt that Khalil Abdul Mustafa had a life-affirming impact on Butch Anthony. Whether it was Khalil's charismatic personality, the power of Islam, or just the right moment to reach Butch spiritually, the confluence of events worked, and the incorrigible shoplifter and drug addict was reborn. There would still be setbacks and obstacles to over-come—criminal acts and drugs were not instantaneously eradicated from his life—but there was now purpose, understanding, and the semblance of a moral compass that had never been there before. Butch still had a long way to travel, but at least now he knew the direction back; there was a path to follow.

During the two months he celled with Khalil, Butch absorbed more than he thought he was ever capable of understanding. He started to prac-tice *salat,* or pray five times a day, read as much as he could get his hands on, digest an array of Arabic terms and concepts, and dream of one day making a *hajj,* or pilgrimage to Mecca. Pleased and uplifted by the changes he saw in himself, he asked Khalil to perform the same spiritual guidance for the other men on the block. Khalil's answer stunned him. He said that Butch should do it himself. He wanted Butch to become Allah's agent in the prison.

Butch laughed in disbelief at the ridiculous suggestion. He felt he was in no way prepared for such an undertaking. He was a student himself, a neophyte still learning the basic tenets of a foreign religion. Khalil assured him that he was capable of the task and further argued that he would be leaving soon, going home; it would be up to Butch to carry on Allah's work in the jail.

Not long thereafter, the day of Khalil's departure arrived. Butch had mixed emotions. His friend and mentor was leaving and he was happy for him, but there was still so much to learn. Who would provide the necessary instruction? Moreover, Butch felt a cloud of insecurity hanging over him. Khalil had given him an anchor, an anvil of stability, answering all his questions logically, documenting them historically, putting his doubts to rest. Now he'd have to educate himself, while at the same time trying to create the same supportive and reassuring religious atmosphere for others that Khalil had provided for him.

Butch and Khalil gave each other a long hug and wished each other a successful life. As they said their goodbyes, Butch realized that in all the years he had spent in prison, he had never gotten this close to anyone. Khalil had opened him up to a new life, a spiritual life. As long as Khalil was around, peace pervaded the cell.

But now he was gone. Though unsure he could carry it off, Butch went about his task in a businesslike manner. He shunned prison drugs and took no part in jailhouse pranks, tried to carry himself with dignity, and encouraged others to take part in the correctional system's more meaningful educational programs. He also cautioned newcomers about the medical research studies. Yes, they were the only way an inmate could earn a buck while in jail, but the potential repercussions could be devastating.

Butch continued to educate himself. He read a wide array of material, spent hours in the prison's meager library, and sought to help others who inquired about Islam. He also investigated the possibility of procuring a Koran. As far as he was aware, custodial authorities had never let the bible of Islam inside the House of Correction. It was a goal he would become fixated on.

One of his first challenges came in the form of the Nation of Islam. They were unaccustomed to religious competition in prison, especially regarding matters of Islamic interpretation, and Butch Anthony had appeared on their radar screen. It was a dangerous place to be. Converts to orthodox Islam presented a threat, one that they well knew how to eliminate.

"In dealing with the Nation of Islam," says Butch, "you had to be very selective in what words you used. If they interpreted anything you said as an insult, they'd kill your ass. The Fruit of Islam could really be vicious, and everybody on the street or in jail damn well knew it. They were very protective of Elijah Muhammad and didn't want to hear anything bad about him.

"I had become a problem for them. They knew I was offering another brand of Islam in the jail. They weren't happy.

"They came to my cell one morning. There were six or seven of them. I recognized a few of them. They were in jail for some serious stuff and givin' me some stern looks. I knew I was in trouble."

"We hear you're callin' yourself a Muslim," said one of the men threateningly.

"That's right, I'm a convert to Islam," Butch replied.

"Is that so? Well, we been hearin' some stuff about you and it ain't good. We ain't leaving this here cell until we hear you say there is no other God but Allah and the Honorable Elijah Muhammad is his prophet."

Though he knew that his life was in danger, Butch didn't waver.

"You're asking the impossible of me," he replied. "You all better get your beds and move them in here, because I will not say that. That's blasphemy."

"Why's that?" said one of the men.

"That's too bad for you, motherfucker," said another.

The men stepped closer. Butch could not only smell the strong scent of garlic on their breath but could feel the testosterone and evil intent. He was certain blood was about to be spilled.

"Listen, I'm not out to offend you or the Nation of Islam," Butch said quickly. "I will say that Elijah Muhammad is a messenger of God, but I won't say he's a prophet. That would be blasphemy. I won't do it."

There was a long moment of uncomfortable silence. Butch braced himself. He felt the inevitable coming. Then one of the FOI spoke up and said, "Yeah, I guess that's all right. That's good enough. But if we catch you badmouthing the Honorable Elijah Muhammad, you won't be so lucky next time."

The men left Butch's cell as quickly as they had appeared. He knew he had dodged a serious beating, maybe worse.

"I really expected I was gonna get fucked up," recalls Butch of that tense time. "The joint was loaded with Black Muslims, and I was the only one teaching Sunni Islam. There were a few times that I thought they were gonna do me in, but they didn't. I was surprised. They basically left me alone."

"My Spiritual Awakening"

143

Butch Anthony's conversion to Islam not only ruffled the feathers of the followers of Elijah Muhammad; his actions also caught the attention of prison administrators. In fact, he sought them out; he wanted something from them—permission to bring a Koran into the jail.

If other religious groups were allowed to have Bibles, Butch reasoned, it seemed only fair that adherents of Islam should be able to gain access to their bible, the Koran. He contacted his mother and asked her to send him a Koran. For a devout southern Baptist, the request would normally have been anathema, but Mrs. Anthony appreciated small wonders, especially those affecting her crime-prone and drug-addicted son. Like Laura, Butch's ex-wife, Mrs. Anthony had been receiving startlingly positive and spiritually uplifting letters from her son. He seemed to have rejected illicit drugs and sworn off the prison experiments, and he wrote movingly of turning his life around. She must have said to herself, "Anything that can help that boy is good. I don't care what it is; if it helps him, I'll try it." She would have sung hallelujah in Arabic if she had known the language.

Butch asked her to go to Robin's Book Store on 13th Street. He was fairly sure that the store, which was known for its progressive politics and for sending books into prisons, would either have a Koran for sale or be able to get one. Weeks went by. After waiting nearly two months and hearing assurances from his mother that she had carried out her task, Butch decided to confront the authorities. He turned in a request slip to see his social worker.

Two days later he received a corridor pass. Determined, but intent on being diplomatic, he wanted answers as to why the Koran had not arrived. When he was finally escorted into the prison's social service unit, he was led to a desk where a short white man in his early thirties was shuffling papers and talking on the telephone.

"Mr. Anthony," he said, after hanging up the phone, "have a seat. You put a request in to see me. What can I do for you?"

"I've come to see you about some literature that was sent to me. I never received it. It's been nearly two months. I want know what happened to it."

The social worker sat back in his chair and sighed.

"There's a prison policy, Mr. Anthony," said the social worker, "that we're not going to be able to get around. We don't allow Korans into the prison. Over the years the book has been the source of disturbances and in some cases riots. The book is restricted. We don't let it inside anymore. We'll give it to you on your way out of the institution."

Frustrated, but maintaining his composure, Butch argued that there were Seventh-Day Adventists, Jehovah's Witnesses, Episcopalians, Pentecostals, Catholics, and all sorts of other groups coming into the institution on a regular basis to conduct religious classes, and all of them came in carrying the Bible. Islam, he argued, was a legitimate spiritual faith practiced by millions of people around the world, and Muslims in the Philadelphia Prison System were entitled to their bible as well. "We have a right," concluded Butch, "to have our good book too."

The social worker leaned forward and said, "What kind of Muslim are you, Mr. Anthony?"

"There's only one kind of Muslim," said Butch firmly.

"Are you a Black Muslim?" asked the social worker warily. "Are you a follower of Elijah Muhammad?"

"No," Butch replied firmly. "There's only one kind of Muslim. Anything other than what was taught by the Prophet Muhammad and written in the Koran is blasphemy. Followers of Islam should have the right to have our own religious book."

"I understand how you could feel discriminated against, Mr. Anthony. And I believe you are serious about your religion, but we're not allowed to let Korans into the institution. Why don't you go see the prison librarian and see if he can get one in here for you."

"You know that ain't gonna happen," said Butch. "Hell, the librarian has even less influence in here than you do. He ain't gonna stick his neck out for us. That's why I was willing to use my own money to get one in here."

"Okay, I hear you," said the skeptical social worker. "Let me see what I can do."

As Butch left the social service unit with little to show for his effort, he contemplated what else he could do to leverage a Koran from the authorities. A petition signed by fellow inmates, letters to elected officials, and a few other notions came to mind. Sleepless a good portion of the night, he wondered how he could have improved his session with the social worker, what better arguments he could have made, and what a more expansive and impressive vocabulary could have accomplished. Butch was hard on himself; the encounter only confirmed his view that a high school dropout and drug addict could never replace Khalil. It was hopeless.

The next morning Butch was called to the cell block gate; he had received a cardboard package in the mail. It was the Koran his mother had purchased at Robin's Book Store months earlier. To his knowledge, he was the first inmate in many years to gain possession of a Koran in the House of Correction.

Though the event wasn't worthy of a *New York Times* article, it did attract notice in the institution. Even the Nation of Islam was impressed by Butch's coup, and in fact came courting. Butch Anthony's proselytizing had already caught their attention, but he now had to be shown a good deal more deference. He had not only obtained a Koran, he had procured it from the authorities. The Nation of Islam even sent a delegation to his cell. They wanted to borrow the book overnight. Their tone was far more conciliatory than it had been on their earlier visit. Though technically an organizational competitor, he had pulled off something they had been unable to do.

Butch was becoming somebody in the jail. Islam was transforming him from an addict with no future into a man with a purpose who preached the Koran, read widely, and studied an array of issues and subjects. No longer a needle-craving deadbeat or a guinea pig for hire, he was now somebody to be reckoned with.

Much like the Nation of Islam and other proselytizing religious sects looking to increase their numbers, Butch sought new converts among those coming into the institution. Though he was reasonably successful, he learned that many subscribers were "jailhouse Muslims," men for whom conversion was of short duration and strictly tied to their period of incarceration. Newcomers to imprisonment were receptive to anyone or any philosophy that appeared friendly. Protection in whatever form was most desirable. Butch did not take offense at this. He understood the jail dynamic as well as anyone and tried to cultivate the truly sincere. His intention, as he said, was to do "the right thing."

Seeking out others like himself who were serious about their conversion to Islam, Butch formed a tight nucleus with several inmates to practice and propagate their faith. One of them was Vincent Peas—now known as Abdul Rahman—who had been a practicing Muslim for years. Butch was determined to learn as much as he could. One day, in a small but reverent ceremony in the corner of the prison yard, Rahman, along with four other Muslim brothers acting as official witnesses, gave Butch a new name, his Sunni Muslim name. A special *shahada,* or Islamic oath, was crafted for the occasion. Brother Butch would now be known as Yusef, the Muslim equivalent of Joseph, or *he who adds beauty and perfection to the world.* Though they were small in number and sequestered in a crowded and raucous prison exercise yard, Butch was impressed with the importance of the event, the meaning of his new Islamic name, and the history and significance of the declaration of faith he had just made.

As Yusef he practiced *salat,* praying five times each day, tried to carry himself with dignity at all times, and followed the teachings of Muhammad. The transformation was nothing short of remarkable, and others took notice. Gradually others would join the nascent Islamic movement, and many of the new converts came from the ranks of the Nation of Islam.

As Butch now recalls, "A lotta guys were leaving the Black Muslims for Sunni Islam. The truth of what we were saying was pulling them in. They were leaving the drills, the marching, and the hate of the Nation for the beauty of pure Islam. It was the real thing."

Butch, or Yusef, as he was being called more and more, took pride in such cell block triumphs, as well as in his own personal transformation. No longer a dumb jitterbug looking to get high or involved in foolish jailhouse stunts, he was now sober, a seeker of knowledge, a man dedicated to the principles of Islam.

147

"It Was a *Jihad*"

In a matter of months Yusef had completed his sentence. Once again he left the House of Correction, or "the Creek," as the inmates and guards called the medium-security facility on Pennypack Creek, with an air of excitement. The anticipation of freedom was there as usual, but this time the prospect of a new, righteous life accompanied him back out onto the street. Edward Anthony had made vast strides in turning his life around during this last prison stint, but the old siren call of the streets would prove too strong to resist. Unfortunately, he was still more Butch than Yusef.

The evening of his release, Butch was invited to an impromptu party held in his honor. His old friends and their addictive behavior were prominently on display. An assortment of alcoholic beverages, marijuana, and heroin were the party items du jour. As Butch willingly concedes, he hadn't "reached that level where religion was strong enough" to overcome his bad habits when presented with such temptations. The pull of drugs and a petty criminal lifestyle to support his habit were overwhelming. His process of spiritual conversion was still in its early stages. Though he would take issue with the characterization, Butch, it turned out, wasn't much more than a jailhouse Muslim himself.

Almost immediately he was back boosting sweaters from clothing stores and chunks of beef from food markets throughout Philadelphia. All the old habits returned, although, during his more lucid moments, Butch could hold listeners' attention when discussing the merits of Islam, the importance of *salat,* and his desire to be known by his Muslim name. His friends took notice; Butch had never spoken of religion before. But these periods of sober reflection and talk of divine guidance were fleeting, and then the old, directionless,

13

drug-addled Butch would return. Where would he score his next quart of wine, bottle of cough syrup, or shot of heroin?

It wasn't long before Butch was nailed on a technical violation. His parole was revoked and he was returned to the county jail he had come to know so well. His three months on the street were one of his smallest windows of freedom yet. Embarrassed and disgusted with himself as he sat with the other derelicts in a noisy, crowded Detention Center dormitory, he couldn't help but realize that he had become one of those lost souls he had seen a decade before, on his initial trip through the Philly prisons. Dazed, foul-smelling winos and drug addicts who spent their life chasing a high and going in and out of prison, men without pasts, hope, or futures: Butch was one of them.

Within a week he was shipped from the DC to Holmesburg Prison. He was mildly surprised, in that Holmesburg was usually reserved for the system's worst offenders, the killers, rapists, and violent assaulters, who had bail set high and needed a thirty-five-foot wall to keep them in. Butch saw his transfer to the toughest joint in the city as an additional penalty for his inability to survive in the free world without breaking the law.

Though a small-time criminal player, Butch knew many of the Burg's residents. He was as much at home here as he was in his North Philly neighborhood. The constant yelling and screaming that echoed through the cell blocks, the bandaged inmates participating in patch tests, and the pervasive gloom of the dilapidated nineteenth-century structure were both familiar and revolting. He had made his bed, and now he had to sleep in it.

Once again behind bars, Butch tried to set a course that would keep him safe and out of harm's way. The medical research program was definitely out. Fooling around with the other brothers on the block and getting into trouble was also out. But furthering his education was something worth looking into. And that went double for his religious studies. Islam was one of the few things providing him with a degree of psychological comfort and satisfaction at this point.

"The Burg was a wild, dangerous joint," recalls Butch, "and if you didn't keep your head straight you could easily lose your mind. The noise, the violence, the games people played on each other was enough to drive you crazy. Throw in corrupt guards, those weird experiments, predatory gangs that roamed the jail, and the fierce competition for new members between Black Muslims and orthodox Muslims, and you're ready for a nervous breakdown.

"I threw myself back into Islam and tried to learn as much as I could. I hung around with guys who knew more than I did, read a lot, and went to all the prayer services, particularly *juma* on Friday afternoons, when an imam from the streets would come in to lead the service. Things were bad at the Burg. The brothers practicing Islam were hardly getting any of the things that other religions were getting. They were really getting worked up about it. I was able to get more from the administration at the Creek than all these more experienced brothers were getting at Holmesburg. Yeah, I knew Holmesburg was a bad joint and required more security and safety precautions, but they were really blocking the practice of our religion."

Unbeknownst to Butch, however, something was in the works that was designed to redress the growing laundry list of perceived slights, constant negativity, and discriminatory policies perpetuated by the prison authorities. It was something that would result in bloodshed and the loss of life. It would also capture news headlines around the country.

As a recently arrived inmate at Holmesburg, Butch didn't comprehend the level of anger that was brewing or exactly what was in the making, but he realized in retrospect that something unusual was afoot. One incident in particular stands out in his mind, though he passed it off at the time as a simple misunderstanding due to his incomplete knowledge of Islamic prayer services. On a Friday afternoon in late May 1973, just after the weekly *juma* service, when men were milling about and going back to their respective cell blocks, Butch was pulled into another *salat*—a special *salat*. An additional prayer after the normal *juma* service was highly unusual, but Butch didn't argue or question anyone about it.

"They just grabbed me by the arm and pulled me into another *salat*," he recalls. "I didn't know exactly what this additional prayer service was for. There were only a few guys involved in the prayer, but I always tried to show my devotion to Allah. I wanted to learn as much as I could and thought maybe they were honoring me for being so sincere about my religious education."

There may have been another reason Butch didn't question his seemingly more observant Islamic brothers. They were some of the most feared criminals in the jail. Two of the men were particularly celebrated for their ruthlessness; they had killed Philadelphia police officers.

Joseph "Jo-Jo" Bowen was a twenty-six-year-old career criminal who had been convicted of killing Patrolman Joseph Kelly in the Roxborough section of the city in February 1971. Frederick "Bellagoon" Burton, twenty-five, had been convicted of the murder of Sergeant Frank Von Colln Jr., a Fairmount Park guard, several years earlier. Though not particularly impressive physically, Bowen and Burton were feared. They "had bodies"—they had killed people. Housed on a different cell block, Butch only saw them at *juma*, where they acted as Muslim security. Though they were both "thin and seemingly docile," Butch could see that "they were serious about their religion." He could also see how other inmates deferred to them; their reputations preceded them. They were not to be taken lightly, and everyone in the jail knew it.

"I had just started performing the *salat* with the other four men," recalls Butch, "when the imam grabs me by the arm, pulls me into the corridor, and asks me what I'm doing. I told him I was performing a *salat* with the other men. I said, 'They pulled me into this special prayer,' when he just cut me off and scolded me. He was very stern. You could see he was angry. He told me I was never to join those men again in such a service. I had no idea what was up and just wrote it off as something I did wrong due to my lack of knowledge of Islamic prayer practices. Once again, my ignorance had gotten in the way."

Butch left the *juma* service and didn't think of the incident again. Two days later he was called down to center and notified he was being discharged. Though he had no idea why he was being released early, he was overjoyed. He had been at his mother's house only two days when he heard the shocking news one afternoon on television—the warden and deputy warden of Holmesburg Prison had been murdered in cold blood. The breathless network commentator, breaking in on one of his mother's favorite soap operas, announced that Warden Patrick N. Curran, forty-seven, and Deputy Warden Robert F. Fromhold, fifty-one, had just been brutally murdered at Holmesburg Prison during an inmate uprising. Another officer, Captain Leroy Taylor, had been severely wounded and was being treated at a local hospital.

Butch was stunned. He began switching channels, searching other local television stations for additional news, and learned that there had been a "confrontation with Muslim activists" and "a bloodletting involving Islamic prisoners." Throughout the afternoon and evening, as local and national news agencies pieced together the bloody story—and what was proclaimed to be the first murder of a warden and deputy warden ever to take place in an American prison—Butch gradually understood the ominous nature of that special *salat* he had been part of just a few days earlier.

When the names of the perpetrators were announced—Frederick Burton and Joseph Bowen—his suspicions were confirmed.

"Damn. Incredible," he said to no one in particular as he sat glued to the TV screen. "They really killed those guys. It was a *jihad*."

His Islamic brothers had become so distraught and so filled with anger at being deprived of the freedoms enjoyed by more mainstream religions prison groups that they had taken up arms. The *salat* he had been momentarily pulled into days earlier was a special prayer for those preparing for a struggle, a *jihad*. Newspaper reports over the following days described the death struggle, the blood-splattered walls, accounts of Curran and Fromhold being repeatedly stabbed by monomaniacal prisoners, and the murderous careers of the two perpetrators.

According to eyewitness accounts, Burton and Bowen had been granted a meeting with Deputy Warden Fromhold to air their complaints regarding the second-class status of orthodox Muslims in the jail. The discussion became heated almost immediately and quickly turned violent, as both inmates set upon the prison official. Though it was unclear whether the inmates had brought shanks with them or managed to get to the stash of confiscated homemade weapons kept in the deputy warden's desk, Fromhold was soon fighting for his life. Hearing the commotion from across the hall, Warden Curran rushed to his deputy's aid, only to be stabbed repeatedly as well. By the time Captain Taylor and other officers entered the now blood-covered office and subdued the inmates, Fromhold and Curran were taking their last breaths. Both men were pronounced dead on arrival at Northeast Philadelphia's Nazareth Hospital.

153

Butch cringed at the thought that he had nearly been part of that maelstrom of violence. He also shuddered at the thought of what life must now be like on the Holmesburg cell blocks in the aftermath of the murders. Just contemplating the retribution being meted out to his Muslim brothers by vengeful guards chilled him. Never a walk in the park, Holmesburg must now be a literal hell on earth. He reflected on how lucky he was to have been pulled out of the *salat* by the imam, and to have been released early. He wasn't used to such good fortune. But he could not rid his mind of images of the bloody struggle in the deputy warden's office and the subsequent revenge by correctional officers. Butch was conflicted, feeling both fortunate and guilty.

As the Philadelphia media played up every angle of the gruesome and unprecedented story, he dealt with his psychic pain as he normally did—by medicating himself with street drugs. His friends were all experienced Holmesburg hands, and the murders were the talk of the neighborhood. Known now by many as Yusef, a sometime practicing Muslim, Butch was repeatedly quizzed on what had gone down in the jail. His inability to give more than strained and unconvincing explanations of how a peace-loving religion had resulted in such bloodshed only deepened his need for chemical escape. The next forty-eight hours were a blur of alcohol and drugs. This concerted effort to outrun reality would lead to some of the most terrifying and dramatic events of his life.

Along with two friends, Leon Washington and John Mason, Butch drank and doped himself into oblivion. As the booze and dope ran out, however, they started to fret and argue about where the next bottle of wine or bag of heroin would come from. The notion of earning money to buy what they needed was quickly scuttled. Washington and Mason were so devoid of logic by this point that they were determined to get what they needed by any means necessary. They cooked up a bold plan to rip off a small-time neighborhood drug dealer who sold the product out of his house. Butch was hesitant, as strong-arm tactics had never been his MO, and the intended victim was a family acquaintance. But his reluctance was no match for his need for a fix and the peer pressure of Washington and Mason. The three men went to the dealer's house at 27th and Susquehanna and found they were in luck: Sol, the owner, was out and had left his home and business in the hands of youthful caretaker named Stan. Butch wanted to stay outside as the lookout, but his friends would have none of it. "You don't come in," yelled Mason, "then you don't get none of the goods, motherfucker."

The young man who mistakenly opened the door was quickly overpowered by the three stick-carrying assailants, tied to a chair, and forced to disclose the location of the drugs. Though six bundles of heroin were discovered, Mason felt there should have been more and started threatening Stan with a serious beating. He then began to search the house. Butch argued that they had more than enough dope for the three of them and should get out while the going was good. He grew increasingly nervous as Mason started to bag shirts and pants from closets and drawers; he was taking everything he could get his hands on. When he saw Mason grab a Koran from a nightstand, he decided he had had enough. He told Mason that things had gone too far and that they should just take the drugs and go. He said he wanted no part of stealing anyone's clothes or Koran.

Butch was adamant; they should just get out before Stan came home. The lecture worked, and the three men exited the house with several thousand dollars' worth of heroin.

For the next three days, Washington, Mason, and Anthony partied hard. Six bundles—twenty-five bags to a bundle—represented a veritable gold mine to the three junkies. Some was sold or given away, but most of the heroin went into their arms and those of their friends who came to share in the ill-gotten goods. It was a good time. But good times don't last forever, and that was especially true for Edward "Butch" Anthony.

"I was sleeping on the living room couch at my mother's house," recalls Anthony, "when the phone rang. I heard my brother Wilbert pick it up. All I heard him say was, 'Oh man. He did what? Are you kidding me?' 'Oh man, damn, how much? That dumb son of a bitch.' I figured it was Stan calling, since he and my brother were friends. I knew they were talking about me.

"I made pretend I was asleep, and my brother just walked out of the house cursing me every step of the way. I figured I was in trouble, but I didn't really know how bad things would get. When I got up and left the house a little while later, I had just stepped out on the street when a guy from the neighborhood comes running up to me and says, 'Butch Anthony. Whadja do now, you dumb nigger? You better be watchin' your back. Those bow-tie-wearing motherfuckers are looking for your black ass.' I asked him what the hell he was talking about and he said that a carload of nasty-lookin' Black Muslims were traveling around North Philly asking about me. It gave me a chill, but the scariest thing may have been hearing that they had a picture of me and were showing it to everybody, trying to find out where I lived and hung out.

"Man, I didn't know what the hell to do. I knew those guys didn't play around. I needed to get off the street as quickly as possible. I made a few phone calls and heard it was all true. The brothers from the Nation of Islam had put a contract out on me. Apparently the stash of drugs Stan was holding was theirs, and now they were showing a photograph of me that Stan had given them. Man, I was scared to death. I didn't know who to trust. They killed people for a lot less than what I had done. I knew I was a dead man for sure if they found me."

Butch was afraid to leave his mother's house, and on those rare occasions when he did, he was afraid to return, fearing the Muslims had the house staked out and would be waiting to pounce. He was forced to return after dark and by circuitous routes that had him jumping over backyard fences, sneaking through unlit alleyways, and taking any other well-hidden path he could contrive. Butch even spotted some wanted posters of him tacked on neighborhood telephone poles. The gravity of the situation only increased when Wilbert Anthony offered to pay Stan a lump sum of money for the stolen drugs, only to learn that the Nation of Islam wouldn't rescind the contract placed on his brother's head. They wanted to teach him and others a lesson. Butch needed to get out of town, but he couldn't—he had no money.

"I was desperate," says Butch. "The only thing I could think of was to go into the orthodox Muslim mosque at 19th and Montgomery. I was hoping they wouldn't find me, or at least would leave me alone if I was hanging out at the mosque of another religious group. Masjid Muhajadeen was a converted horse stable that was continually being rehabbed and expanded. They now had big, beautiful Persian rugs, newly painted rooms, and the entire place was kept very clean. There were new converts all the time, and they were now drawing as many as 250 people for a *juma* service and Islamic holidays. I also knew there were some Muslim brothers that were actually living there. They were *khuddaam (al-masjid)*, individuals who leave their homes to serve the *masjid*. Yeah, a lot of them were homeless or had other problems, but it was a way for them to get a roof over their heads and straighten their lives out. I went over to the mosque and talked to Ali Ahmed, the imam of the mosque. He was like me, in his midthirties, and had seen me come for *juma* services periodically. Fortunately, he hadn't heard about anything that was going down on the street. I told him a story about me wanting a new life and my desire to serve Allah and the mosque. He didn't give me a yes or no at that time, but just said he'd think about it and give me a call."

Butch went back to his mother's house and rarely left the premises. The threat of the Black Muslim hit squads, along with the slow, painful ordeal of drug withdrawal, would normally have culminated in an overwhelming desire for his next shot of heroin. Butch never handled pressure well. But searching the neighborhood for a bag of smack now was the equivalent of suicide. He was forced to go cold turkey on his mother's living room couch. He was taking valiums and painkillers, drinking wine, and indulging in anything else he could find in his mother's house to mute the pain of withdrawal.

The call came two days later. Imam Ali Ahmed said Butch could come live at the mosque. Butch packed his few things and immediately went to the Islamic mosque. He was directed to a small bed in communal quarters that housed ten other men and was assigned an assortment of janitorial duties. Cleaning and mopping halls, dusting furniture, and taking out the trash weren't the most rewarding endeavors, but Butch wasn't averse to hard work, and the mosque had become an oasis of security, a safe house. In addition, the mosque began to provide the intellectual and spiritual sustenance that Butch had first been exposed to in the Philadelphia Prison System and now found particularly nurturing. He was forced to "act right, pray five times a day, discuss aspects of the Koran with knowledgeable practitioners, and feel part of something positive."

As the weeks passed, Butch grew increasingly positive not only about himself but about life in general. Optimism once again started to take hold. He learned that the Black Muslims had rescinded the contract on his life after his brother Wilbert paid them for the stolen dope, and his mother was even pleased with her son's new housing arrangements and lifestyle. Islam was totally foreign to her and she put no spiritual stock in it, but if it straightened her son out and kept him out of trouble, it was all right with her. As she told her friends, "If it gives my boy a chance to live one more day, I can live with it."

In short, everything was looking much better for Butch. It was a bad sign.

157

"Feeling Death Blow Past My Face"

"I was finally off of drugs and doing real well," Butch recalls of his initial weeks in the North Philadelphia mosque. "I kicked drugs because I was hemmed in. I had no other choice. I always wanted to kick my drug habit, but never had the strength. Now I not only wasn't able to go out on the street looking for a fix, but was finally in a community that helped me. It was an environment of support and encouragement. Even in prison, guys could get drugs and get high, but in the mosque it was completely forbidden. Any hint of illicit drugs and you were thrown right out. Now I was getting knowledge instead of a heroin high.

"As a *khadim* I was given all sorts of maintenance and custodial work to do. I'd get up in the morning, unlock the front doors of the mosque, vacuum and clean all the rooms, take out the trash, and even did some cooking. The imam took notice of how hard I worked and how appreciative I was that he allowed me to live there. He started giving me some additional duties and assignments that the other guys didn't receive; he was entrusting me with greater responsibility. I was made the *waqil*, or caretaker, and given the keys to the place. I was really pleased. It was a completely new life for me, and I was feeling pretty good.

"Then, about a month into my stay, some little red dots started to appear on my hands. I tried not to give it a thought and kept busy. I didn't want to think anything was happening again. But each day there'd be a few more dots, and some of them were becoming elevated; they were bumps now.

"Then the itching began. It drove me nuts. I'd be rubbing and scratching my hands all day without any relief. I put different lotions and salves on my hands, but nothing seemed to work. Next thing I know, my feet start to break out with these red dots and bumps.

14

I couldn't hide it from myself any longer; this here shit I first got in prison had come back again. It was just like in Holmesburg. Those damn prison experiments had messed me up for good. I thought to myself, I'll never get rid of this shit. I'm gonna be cursed with it the rest of my life.

"The itching was so intense, the only way I could get relief was to run scalding hot water on my hands and feet. Just like back in the prison, when I would stand under a steaming hot shower. People thought I was crazy. But it was the only thing that seemed to help with the pain and itching. I really started to worry and get depressed when the bumps started to fill with pus. When I scratched my hands or feet to relieve the itching, the pustules would break open and this pus-filled fluid would leak out. It was really sickening. It was like ten years earlier when I was back at Holmesburg.

"A couple times the imam must have seen me scratching my hands, and he gave me money to go down to the pharmacy and buy some over-the-counter ointment or salve for the problem. I did, but nothing I bought worked. I was using everything I could find for skin rashes, but the result was the same. I had a whole cabinet full of stuff that wasn't doing a thing. Determined not to let it all affect me, I kept working my various jobs in the mosque. After a while, though, I had to give up working in the kitchen. Handling things like onions, potatoes, and garlic just seemed to aggravate the condition. My hands really became inflamed. Besides, the other guys saw my hands and knew I had something bad. They weren't like the brothers in Holmesburg who thought I had some dread disease and forced me to stop eating with them, but you could see they were concerned. I had to stop cooking for the guys.

"Over the next few weeks things only got worse. My hands and feet started to swell. It was gradual but unmistakable—my hands and feet were swelling up. The other khuddaam at the mosque tried to be helpful, offered me assistance, and did some of my chores around the building. They knew it wasn't like me to be a slacker and lay down on my assignments, but they could see what was going on. It was getting more and more difficult to do things. I was having trouble holding things, and just walking was becoming difficult. It was obvious what some of them were thinking. They'd see me holding my hands under burning hot water and probably say to themselves, 'Man, that cat's a mess.'

"The other khuddaam tried to be as supportive as possible. They asked me all kinds of questions about what I had, when and where I got it, and wasn't there anything I could do about it. When they heard it started with the prison experiments, they said I should get a lawyer and sue someone, but I told them I couldn't, I had signed my rights away. I explained that when you got on these tests they made you sign a waiver saying if anything went wrong, it was on you. I said all of us in jail were desperate for money back then, and the Penn research studies were the best things going. But you could get really fucked up on them. And now I was paying for it big time."

Seeing that he was noticeably impaired, the imam ordered Yusef to see a doctor, only to be told, "I can't. I don't have a medical card or any insurance to pay for a doctor's visit."

The imam scolded Yusef. He told him he needed to see a doctor and then gave him money to cover the cost of the visit and any medication that might be needed. Yusef went to a neighborhood doctor at 31st and Diamond who examined him and prescribed a couple of salves. Though he applied the lotions as instructed, they had no noticeable effect. His hands and feet continued to swell. In fact, as time passed, the problem only grew worse, as his hands and feet began to leach a tremendous amount of moisture. If that wasn't embarrassing enough, his burgeoning extremities also began to emit a foul odor.

Yusef struggled to carry out his chores, and made a concerted effort to hide his increasingly deformed hands and feet, but his health problem was becoming critical. As he recalls, "I couldn't perform *salat* anymore. I couldn't get down on my hands and knees. I had to sit in a chair like the old people do and just lower my head. My hands and feet really started to stink, and they sweat so bad that guys were buying me packages of socks every day, five and six to a package, cause I had to throw the socks out after only wearing them one time. They were ruined, and no amount of washing would rehabilitate them. When I walked, you could hear a squishing noise inside my shoes. My feet were soaking wet. All the time."

His overall health declining rapidly, Yusef could no longer carry out his duties or hide the seriousness of his problem. One morning while working in his office, Imam Ali became distracted by a strange smell. As he searched for the origin of the foul odor, he came upon Yusef, who seemed to be dozing in a chair. "Is that you, Yusef?" asked the imam. "Is that you smelling so bad?"

There was no response. Yusef wasn't dozing; he was nearly unconscious.

"My God, man, look at your hands," said the startled imam as he examined his *khadim* more closely.

Still getting no response, he lifted Yusef's head up. His forehead was extremely warm and his pupils were severely bloodshot. The dark rings around his eyes made him look like a raccoon. His skin tone was now more gray than brown, and his tongue was practically white.

Alarmed, Imam Ali called some *khuddaam* for assistance. They carried their sick colleague back to his bed and Ali got on the phone and called the only number he had for the Anthony family. He informed them that Yusef was very ill. He was running a high fever and should probably go to the hospital. Peasie, Yusef's sister, said she would be right over to help take him to the hospital. While waiting for Yusef's sister to arrive, the imam and *khuddaam* tried to clean and dress their disabled friend. They were all shocked by his condition, and especially by the abnormal size of his hands and feet. It was as if he had elephantiasis. They had a difficult time getting him dressed. His hands were the size of boxing gloves, and it was clearly impossible to put shoes on his feet. The imam sent a *khadim* to the local discount clothing store and told him to buy "the largest pair of slippers or sandals they have." When he came back with a pair of huge 14EEE sandals, they could still only get Yusef's toes into the sandals. He normally wore a size ten-and-a-half shoe.

When his sister Peasie arrived at the mosque with a family brother-in-law and saw her brother, she was horrified. "My God," she screamed, "what the hell did you do to yourself now? Oh my God, you're a mess."

Yusef was in no condition to reply. He couldn't even raise his head. The *khuddaam* helped carry him to the car, and Peasie and the brother-in-law drove as quickly as they could to Philadelphia General Hospital. Though it was a relatively brief journey from North to West Philadelphia, it was still nerve-wracking; Peasie couldn't help reflect on her little brother's recurring travails—the drugs and arrests and repeated incarcerations, and the bizarre, debilitating medical experiments he had undergone. And now this. She didn't know if her brother was cursed or if the whole family was cursed to have such a troubled member. He always seemed to be at death's door.

When they arrived at the hospital's emergency unit, they needed a wheelchair to get him in the building. Once a fine, state-of-the-art medical institution with expert physicians and a solid reputation, PGH was now a tired, run-down city hospital short on staff and supplies, yet overburdened with a steady stream of the city's poorest residents. Yusef was not only not ambulatory; he was near death. Bureaucratic personnel at the reception desk, however, asked for a medical card or other form of insurance coverage.

In addition, there were forms and papers to be filled out. Peasie was both embarrassed and outraged by the delay. Her brother had no health coverage, just a strange malady that was obviously killing him. Couldn't they dispense with the insurance forms for just a moment and attend to her brother's dire condition?

The officious intake personnel continued to ask questions about Yusef as Peasie tried to contain her emotions and move the admittance process along. She was about to burst, when suddenly someone behind her shouted, "Are you out of your damn mind? Can't you see this man is in critical condition? Get this man in the hospital now. You can take care of that paperwork later."

It was a PGH physician in a white lab coat passing through the admittance area. He had noticed Yusef's condition and realized the severity of the situation. There was little time to waste. Yusef was taken immediately to a treatment room where additional medical personnel arrived and quickly started to check his vital signs and examine his terribly swollen hands and feet. The nurses were amazed at the size of his fingernails, which resembled claws.

Yusef, who was falling in and out of consciousness and oblivious to the frenetic activity going on around him, can only recall "feeling death blow past my face."

While giving their patient a series of pills and shots, the doctors also reconfigured a gurney, enabling Yusef to submerge his hands and feet in four large plastic containers that held a therapeutic solution. He and the odd contraption were then wheeled down the corridor, into an elevator, and then up to the fourth floor, where he was immediately undressed and placed in a bathtub filled with warm, chemically treated water.

It was the nurses' good fortune that their patient was incapacitated and barely conscious, for he normally would have screamed bloody murder and never allowed them to do what they were about to do—rip the palms and soles of his hands and feet off.

As Yusef lay in the warm solution, three nurses—two holding his arm steady and one wielding a sharp scalpel—started to cut into his grossly oversized hand. The first incision was made where the palm meets the wrist. As the nurse moved the scalpel along the base of the wrist, there was surprisingly little blood. It was like watching a butcher cut gristle away from a chunk of sirloin. Yusef's hand at this point was more fatback than actual flesh and blood. Once the several-inch incision was made, the

"Feeling Death Blow Past My Face"

nurse grabbed the half-inch-thick flap of petrified meat that was Yusef's palm and started to pull it up and off his hand. Using the scalpel to make strategic cuts at both sides and along each of the fingers, the palm was gradually separated from the rest of the swollen extremity. The nurses holding Yusef's arm steady winced at the unusual procedure, while the debilitated and feverish patient registered what little protest he could muster.

When the nurse had peeled the thick sheath of flab off, a raw, bloody wound remained. It was now more obvious why the procedure was undertaken in a tub of water. They then began to work on Yusef's other hand. Within minutes, two perfectly formed slabs of gristle and flesh in the shape of oversized gloves were lying on the blood-stained linoleum floor, and the green-tinted liquid in the tub gradually turned from pink to crimson.

The patient, sweat pouring off his brow and occasionally delirious, was now pulled more deeply into the tub so that the nurses could grapple with their next task—flaying his feet. Approaching the size of turkey basins, the ugly extremities were a mass of petrified flesh. While her assistants held one leg steady, the nurse with the scalpel began to dig into Yusef's foot between the toes and the base of the sole. Liquid muck poured out with each additional penetrating incision. One nurse had to turn her head away from the grisly sight, as the scalpel proceeded to cut its way through a good half-inch of meat and dead skin. Yusef occasionally whimpered, "Oh God, you're killing me," but it's unlikely that the pain was all that intolerable. Most of his foot was beyond sensation. And besides, Yusef was barely conscious.

As incisions were made along both sides of the foot, the head nurse would periodically pull the thick slab of skin down and off the patient. The nurses were amazed at the size and gross nature of it but refrained from any lengthy commentary, as they hadn't completed their mission. They had another foot to do.

For the fourth time, one of Yusef's limbs was immobilized, deep incisions made, and disgustingly thick dead skin peeled off. Though the taxing, stomach-churning ordeal had left them all tired, sweaty, and blood-spattered, they were still not finished. They now had to treat Yusef's raw and bloody hands and feet with a red ointment and then a purple antiseptic solution to guard against further infection. He was then taken out of the tub, dried off, and set on a gurney, where the red and purple antibacterial solutions were reapplied.

After taking several potent sedatives and other medications for his fever, Yusef quickly fell asleep. He would remain that way for several days.

"I don't know whether I was in a coma or just asleep," says Yusef of those lost days, "but I do know I had some terrible nightmares. I was dreaming all sorts of things. I would remember those fire-and-brimstone speeches by the minister at my mother's church that used to frighten me as a child; going to the local drugstore as a teenager and getting high on cough syrup; and the chill of walking into Holmesburg for the first time. What I really remember having nightmares about were those tests that fucked me up. My body breaking out in a strawberry rash; becoming paranoid and being called 'Outer Limits' by the other inmates when I got on those army tests; and my sister screaming in fear when she saw what the experiments had done to me. That's all I can recall. I don't know if it was a dream, nightmare, or what. But that's all I remember, all that negative stuff."

While Yusef remained incommunicado during those early days in the hospital, a family vigil was held at his bedside. His mother, now in her late seventies, and two of his sisters and their husbands made repeated trips to PGH to visit him. Imam Ali and several *khuddaam* also stopped by periodically. Nearly a week went by before Yusef came to and began to communicate. Sisters Peasie and Lucille and his mother were in the room when he began to interact with visitors.

Exhausted by the trials of her youngest child, Mrs. Anthony was pleased that her son was now conscious and talking, but still ornery enough to let him have it. "Boy," she exclaimed, "you're still trying to kill yourself, aren't you? First it was those drugs and then those damn prison tests. You're determined to kill yourself, aren't you? When are you ever gonna learn?"

Yusef tried to explain to his mother that he hadn't done drugs or taken part in any prison experiments again, but it was no use. He had lost all credibility with her long ago. She was beyond believing anything he said. "I couldn't really blame her," says Yusef. "She always said my lifestyle was irresponsible, and she was right. I was a screwup. And a functional illiterate to boot."

A week had gone by, and though he was no longer at death's door, it would be many more weeks before Yusef was released from the hospital. During that time he was given a steady diet of powerful steroids and other medications to combat his infection and try to bring his terribly swollen limbs back to normal size. Dermatologists, with medical students in tow, would stop by his bedside, discuss his case in highly technical terms, and leave Yusef to ponder what all the medical jargon meant.

Occasionally he was asked to provide his medical history. He explained that his health had always been fine until he participated in the Holmesburg medical studies, but the issue seemed to draw little comment and shed even less light on his current malady. Even the hospital's head dermatologist, who had taken an interest in his case, was at a loss, though he thought his patient's five daily prayer rituals might have a salutary effect. "The doctor told me that performing *salat* may have saved my life," says Yusef. "He said that the poisons that had entered my body were drawn to my most active nerve endings, and gravitational pull during prayer drew these poisons to my hands and feet. If not for that, he said, they would have traveled to my chest cavity and probably killed me."

Yusef was informed he'd have to undergo a series of patch tests—dermatological experiments—to better understand what had happened to him. The thought of more scientific experiments gave him pause; he just shook his head in dismay. He was too weak to object, however, and rationalized that these PGH doctors hadn't been behind the prison experiments. He told himself that they were new, decent doctors trying to help him. He wanted to believe that the new tests were therapeutic in nature and designed to correct what was destroying his health. He ultimately agreed to take part.

Yusef was taken to a dingy basement laboratory where he had a series of patches applied to his back. As the doctors and medical technicians went about their business of putting ointments, liquids, and other foreign substances on gauze pads and then attaching them to his body, Yusef couldn't help but think to himself, "This is how all this shit got started in the first place. These research doctors and their damn patch tests."

The PGH sensitivity studies failed to explain what had caused his skin to erupt or his limbs to swell. All the head dermatologist told him was, "Young man, you're worth a million dollars in medical research. You have A-1 sensitive skin."

Yusef didn't know if he should be proud or ashamed. But as the weeks went by and he continued his daily regimen of pills and injections, and watched nurses swab various potions on his hands and feet, he had time to reflect on his life and his current condition.

He wondered why, out of all the Anthony children, he was the only one to be such a total screwup. His older brother Joe had been an accomplished boxer and traveled around the world with the great Joe Louis, putting on boxing exhibitions during World War II. His sister Edna was a well-liked and appreciated schoolteacher, Peasie was going to school to become a nurse, and his other older brothers, although not professionals, were at least law-abiding citizens and respected members of the community. Why had he been such an embarrassment? Why his need for drugs, why the numerous arrests, why the inexplicable medical conditions? "Why me?" he repeatedly asked himself.

Bedridden for long periods, he also had time to contemplate larger social questions, issues that seemed to affect him and many others like him. If he was some kind of social pariah, a functional illiterate with a chronic drug problem who repeatedly broke the law, why weren't the powers that be doing something to cure him, to rehabilitate him? Putting him in jail obviously wasn't working. And it didn't seem to be working for the hundreds of others he saw each time he was incarcerated. With all the great and creative minds out there, couldn't they think of something more beneficial and productive than locking up troubled people in primitive institutions and giving them little or no positive guidance?

He also began wondering why those medical experiments were being done in the prison system, anyway. Was that supposed to be part of his punishment? And why were healthy people like himself used in strange, obviously dangerous medical research? If science needed test subjects, why weren't they using the many sick people already out there looking for cures? Why were doctors more interested in getting healthy people sick, when there were already enough sick people out there who would be willing to volunteer for experiments? Did imprisoned African Americans like himself have value only as test subjects?

Yusef was never one to buy readily into racist arguments proffered by the likes of the Nation of Islam, but maybe the NOI was right about medical research in prison. Why did incarcerated black people seem to be the backbone of this operation? The more he thought about these questions, the more frustrated and disillusioned he became.

One afternoon when he had been in the hospital for approximately a month, Yusef was paid a visit by Tariq, a member of the mosque. Tariq also brought his fiancée, Isla, who was dressed in a beautiful white *hijab* that covered her from head to foot. Isla managed a health food store in West Philadelphia and hid quietly behind her veil during the visit. As Yusef described his ordeal and his pitifully slow recovery, and tried to conceal his swollen limbs, Isla remained silent but took notice of his discomfort.

"Wow, the sister really made me feel embarrassed," recalls Yusef. "She was in a sparkling white *hijab*, and I was falling apart under the covers. I was in so much pain, and my hands and feet were still weeping. Sweat, liquid, whatever, was just pouring out of them. I really felt miserable. Man,

I was so depressed. I felt that my life was just running out of my hands and feet."

During the visit, an orderly came into the room with his dinner. No more than a couple of minutes had passed when Isla, no longer able to restrain herself, said to Yusef, "My God, that's dirt you're eating. No wonder your blood is filthy. If I were to bring you some food, would you eat it? It would be good *halal* food." Yusef was familiar with *halal* food and said yes, he wouldn't have a problem with that.

The next day Isla returned with a big shopping bag filled with goodies. There was a big, round pumpernickel bread that she proceeded to slice and cover with bananas, honey, and tofu. She said, "This is what you need to eat more of and stop eating that filthy meat they're giving you. Can't you see that stuff is killing you? And if you get a craving for sweets, don't eat candy or any refined sugar. Replace it with some of these sunflower seeds and raisins I brought you."

She introduced him to a number of other edibles in the bag and then proceeded to lecture Yusef on the dos and don'ts of a healthy diet and positive lifestyle. She said he must stop eating all meat products and that he should basically maintain a diet of fruits and vegetables.

As best he could from a hospital bed, Yusef tried to abide by Isla's dietary directives. The results were dramatic. "After three days, they couldn't keep me in bed," Yusef says. "I was up and about and moving all over the place." The swelling went down substantially, the pain and discomfort subsided, his ever-present bowel problem relented, and he started to look and feel better. "The darkness around my eyes cleared up," he says, "and the red dots and bumps that covered parts of my body began to fade. My face was almost back to normal. I couldn't believe it."

Neither could the doctors, especially when they heard the once critically ill patient attribute his miraculous recovery to Isla and her mosque-endorsed "alkaloid diet." Most of the medical staff attributed his rapid improvement to conventional medical care, but even the hospital's top dermatologists were puzzled and somewhat open to giving some of the credit to the dietary changes. As one awestruck doctor said, "If it was up to me, I'd have a mosque built right down in the basement and have your friend provide dietary instructions to our entire kitchen staff."

Over the next couple of days, Yusef's health continued to improve. His release from the hospital imminent, the doctors insisted on some further medical studies. With the prospect of a return to normalcy at hand, Yusef agreed, but one of the tests was terribly painful and seemed a throwback to some of the things he had heard about at Holmesburg. "The doctors seemed preoccupied with my nails," he says. "They had grown out like big, curved claws. The doctors stuck needles in my fingers all around the edges of my nails. They bore in real deep and it hurt like hell. I screamed, 'My God, you're killing me. What the hell are you doing to me?' Christ, I began to feel like Jesus being nailed to the cross."

Without benefit of painkillers or an explanation as to its purpose, Yusef endured the test. The next day, his forty-fifth in PGH, he was released to a half-dozen smiling members of his North Philadelphia mosque.

One who seemed especially pleased by Yusef's return was a woman named Sister Jamillah.

169

"A Righteous Life"

"Getting my health back was like being reborn," says Yusef of his return to the mosque at 19th and Montgomery in the summer of '74. "My hands were still swollen, but not nearly as bad as they had been. The stigma of those sweaty, bloated hands was gone, and I could do a lot of my regular jobs again. I could even shake a person's hand; I didn't have to hide them behind my back when meeting somebody for the first time. Sure, I still had problems; handling anything with a high acid content would irritate my hands and cause them to break out. And I could never put rubber gloves on my hands to do some of the more disgusting janitorial work for the same reason. But all in all I could do most of the things I needed to do around the mosque."

Yusef also took on some additional responsibilities that were not part of his job description. One was especially rewarding—mentoring a young man whose parents belonged to the mosque but were getting divorced. Jaffa was just graduating from grade school and entering junior high. He was bright, inquisitive, and enjoyed hanging around the mosque. His mother, Jamillah, was a recent convert, and both mother and son were excited by the new spiritual life Islam offered. They came to the mosque often, and young Jaffa was quite taken by the language, customs, and artwork. He also took a liking to one *khadim* in particular.

"He was smart little kid," says Yusef, "and we would talk about all sorts of subjects. We talked about the Koran, what it meant to be a Muslim, Muhammad's role in history, and many other things. He just seemed to enjoy hanging around me. And I enjoyed him as well. I never talked about it much, but I always felt guilty about not being a better father to my own kids, so I guess that motivated me to be particularly nice to this little kid. And I have to admit, it was nice being appreciated for it. People seemed to recognize I had

15

developed a good relationship with this kid and often complimented me for taking the time to teach him things about Islam and the operations of the mosque. I guess in a way I became his mentor. It was a real change to get those compliments, because too often, where I came from, my neighborhood and especially in prison, going out of your way to do things for people was considered weak, certainly suspicious. If you did a good thing, you were criticized for it."

One person who took notice of the relationship and often expressed her appreciation was Sister Jamillah. "She was a nice-looking woman," recalls Yusef, "and I was most impressed with her mannerisms and how she carried herself. She was a very serious Sunni Muslim and took her *shahada* to heart. She seemed to be coming into the mosque more and more, and I started to be kidded about it by the other *khuddaam*. 'She's interested in you, man,' they'd be telling me all the time. 'She's looking for a new husband.'

"I told 'em, 'Don't be ridiculous. I don't have any money and I'm not even getting a welfare check. How am I gonna marry anyone?'

"It didn't make any difference to 'em. They'd just say, 'Yusef, that sister really digs you.'"

Though Yusef may have been the last one to realize it, Jamillah had indeed taken an interest in him. Her visits became more frequent, and though their initial discussions focused on her son, they soon moved on to more personal subjects, such as her disappointment with local men and her likely relocation to North Carolina.

"She would occasionally talk about the brothers in the mosque," says Yusef, "and the sorry state of marriage material that existed there. She said she was planning to move back south where she had family. I remember on this one occasion I told her not to be so quick to write off the brothers, there were still some good men around. I told her, just be patient, Allah will bring you someone. She turned around as she was leaving the office and with a smile on her face said, 'There's only one brother in this here mosque I would take a chance on and I think he knows who it is.' That's when I knew. That's when I knew the other brothers were right, she was really interested in me."

Their courtship ran through the late summer and fall of 1974. Yusef was quite happy, and so was his family. Though none of the Anthonys was a Muslim, Yusef's troubled life seemed to have taken a turn for the better, and there was genuine optimism that a corner had been turned and that the worst might be over. Islam appeared to have given Yusef purpose and direction, and Jamillah seemed a fine woman of good moral character—somebody who could keep Yusef on the straight and narrow. Their wedding was a large, beautiful affair. Members of the mosque went all out for one of their own.

Yusef was pleased by his family's acceptance of his new wife and religion, and he distinctly remembers Joe, his oldest brother, taking in the atmosphere of the mosque, the wedding ceremony, and the Islamic rituals, and saying, "This ain't bad. This is okay. This ain't bad at all." It was as ringing an endorsement as one was going to get from the stoical former prizefighter concerning his problem-ridden little brother, his new family, and religion.

Yusef, Jamillah, and Jaffa moved into a first-floor apartment two doors down from the mosque that was owned by a friend and member of the mosque. It had impressive high ceilings and enough space for one of the rooms to be turned into a prayer room. Things were definitely looking up for Yusef, but such episodes of peace and tranquility had been short-lived in the past—and they would be once again.

As long as Yusef was a *khadim* living and working in the mosque, money was never an issue. But now that he was on the street and having to support a wife and stepson, he was presented with new challenges. The imam helped by assisting with paperwork that enabled Yusef to get a monthly welfare check, but it was not enough to sustain them. He did other odd jobs to earn money, including one as a window washer.

But the lack of money wasn't the only problem. Unexpectedly, Jaffa became a considerable headache. "As soon as we got married," says Yusef, "the kid started to show his ass. He wouldn't listen to me anymore. He wouldn't even take out the trash when I told him to. We once had a good relationship, enjoyed each other's company, but now he saw me living and sleeping with his mother and he developed a hell of an attitude. It became a big problem, and the kid's father even got involved. He said, 'Look, tell me when you want Jaffa to do something and I'll tell him to do it.'

"Who the hell wants a situation like that, where I have to go to the kid's father to get him to do something as simple as doing his homework or buying groceries at the store? And Jamillah taking Jaffa's side in these arguments only made it worse. I told her she was always defending him, and making me feel like the kid was her husband, not me. All that shit came up to my neck, and I started feeling like a stranger in my own home. Man, it was bad."

Yusef's tenuous grasp on economic and familial stability only became more uncertain when his window-washing gig presented problems old and new—both particularly frightening. First- and second-story washing contracts in various Philly neighborhoods presented only a modest challenge, but larger projects that took him out of the state revealed a mismatch between worker and assignment. Though the pay was better and the jobs of longer duration, there was one immense hurdle he was unable to overcome: Yusef was afraid of heights. "Working on those five- and six-story commercial buildings in Maryland scared the hell out of me," he says. "The foreman saw I had a problem and told me to stay on the ground and prepare the various equipment and cleaning solutions, but I knew he was unhappy, 'cause he hired me to go up and clean windows. I knew I was probably gonna get fired."

As Yusef began each new day in the expectation that it might be his last, another, equally chilling concern arose—little red dots started to reappear on his hands and feet. "I knew I was getting sick again," Yusef recalls of that unnerving moment. "I guess it was stirring all that water containing various cleaning chemicals that caused me to break out. It was the same old thing—red dots and little bumps. I was scared to do anything. I was healthy and strong, climbing ladders and lifting pails of liquid, but I knew what was coming—I was headed towards a relapse."

The grim prospect of his limbs swelling and another lengthy hospital stay forced him to quit his window-washing job. As he had hoped, the threat to his health gradually dissipated, but the lack of income put further strain on his already troubled home life.

As the problems accrued, the prospect of marital bliss gradually went out the window. "The marriage," says Yusef, "certainly didn't match my ideal of the perfect Islamic union. I struggled with all the new responsibilities, but I was too immature. I could never handle responsibility, and this was another example of it. It just got to a point where I couldn't handle it anymore. I decided to take off my *kufi*, put it in my back pocket, walked across the street, and got a bag of heroin.

"I was feeling terrible about myself," says Yusef of his self-destructive decision to use drugs again. "I felt as if everything was going against me. As hard as I tried, I never succeeded. Even the marriage went south on me. Everything always turned out unlike I thought it would. I knew what it meant to use drugs again, but at the time I needed something to relieve the tension, the stress, and the anxiety I was feeling. Yeah, I felt guilty about taking that first shot, but the dope always made me forget all that negativity in my life."

Yusef's slow, steady slide into serious drug use once again was probably apparent to others, but he rationalized that if he kept himself busy and refrained from displaying the pronounced dozing and nodding characteristic of heroin addicts, he could deceive his wife and others. It worked for a good month, or as long as Jamillah and others collaborated in not recognizing what was so painfully obvious. A dispute over a measly ten dollars brought the charade to an end.

"I usually gave Jamillah whatever little money I made," says Yusef. "Well, one day I asked her for $10, and she says, 'What do you want the money for?' I told her I owed a friend ten bucks and wanted to pay him back. She asked for a name so I gave her one, and she said she'd pay him when she saw him on the street. I said no, that I wanted to give it to him. 'You want that money for drugs, don't you?' she yelled at me. 'You're using drugs again, aren't you? You think I don't know what you been doing.'"

Yusef vehemently denied the charge, but his wife knew him too well. They argued for some time, until Jamillah came out with a declaration that stunned Yusef. "We're supposed to be a couple," she screamed. "We're supposed to share everything, right? If you want to do this to yourself, then I'm gonna do it too. You're gonna have to do it with me."

Astonished, Yusef was unsure that he had heard her correctly, but her demeanor said it all. Jamillah wanted to share the drug experience with her husband. Yusef tried arguing with her, but she was unrelenting. She insisted they share everything, and that included his drug addiction. He would get his fix only if she would get one as well.

Yusef knew that Jamillah had at one time smoked reefer, but she had stopped that long ago and was adamantly opposed to harder drugs like heroin. Despite the significant personal and ethical boundary he was about to cross, Yusef took the $10, went across the street, and bought a bag of dope. When he returned home, Yusef prepared his shot as usual and injected the heroin into his vein while Jamillah looked on nervously. He then rinsed the needle and prepared another solution of considerably less potency for his wife. Then he told her to go and get a string or shoelace to use as a tourniquet. When she left the room, Yusef quickly injected himself a second time and then hurriedly went about making another shot for his wife. This one, though, contained only water. Yusef had no intention of introducing his wife to heroin.

Reluctant, but still determined to share the drug experience with her husband, Jamillah held out her arm. Within seconds of the needle's entering her arm Jamillah began to have heart palpitations, lay back on the sofa, and alarmingly proclaimed she was about to faint. Yusef tried to conceal his laughter but couldn't help himself. "I knew I had given her a water shot," he says, "but she acted like she had been given a double dose and was gonna die. I had to calm her down and tell her it was only a very small dose I had given her and she was gonna be all right, but she had convinced herself it was the real thing. It was so damn funny I couldn't stop laughing. I nearly fell off the sofa."

It would be quite some time before laughter was heard in the Anthony household again. Although that would be Jamillah's first and last experience with a heroin needle, Yusef was about to descend into one of the most painful and humiliating periods of his life.

Little by little, various objects—appliances and clothing—began to go missing from the apartment. One day it was Jamillah's artificial flowers, the next day, the toaster, two days later, the kitchen set. He received $75 for their refrigerator. Yusef's heroin addiction was devouring everything they owned.

Jamillah was torn apart with grief. "I love you," she told her husband, "but you're crazy. You're killing yourself." He was also killing their marriage. Jamillah remained loyal throughout, on some occasions even giving him things to sell so he could buy his next fix. "She was so compassionate," says Yusef. "She showed so much understanding and care. She gave me things to sell so I wouldn't have to be boosting things on the street."

Some in the community were saddened by Yusef's destructive behavior but resigned to seeing another brother from an upstanding black family fall prey to the streets. Others were outraged, especially members of the mosque, who deeply resented Yusef's conduct, as well as his treatment of his wife. They decided to act.

"I came home one day," recalls Yusef, "to find the apartment flooded out. There was water everywhere. There was like an inch or two of water in every room. Jamillah and Jaffa and all their clothes and possessions were gone. It was like a barren apartment, just walls and water-covered floors. I had sold or hocked almost everything we owned.

"When I went outside, I was met by Imam Ali. Word obviously got back to him what I was up to, and he confronted me on the front steps. 'You're a disgrace to the community,' he said. 'You're a *kafar* [apostate]. Your actions have destroyed you, embarrassed your wife, and destroyed your family. You're no longer fit to live with. We've taken your wife out of this wicked lifestyle and placed her with another family. A good family that will take care of her.'

"He warned me," says Yusef, "that if I should try and reach out to her I'd be found in the Schuylkill with my throat slit. He said if I tried to contact her I'd be declared 'legal' according to Islamic law. The meaning was simple. If I fucked around, they'd kill me and throw me in the river."

Yusef defended himself and tried to show that he wasn't intimidated by such threats, but it was all bluster. He was clearly frightened, and rightly so. Though not as vicious as the Nation of Islam, orthodox Muslims could also get physical. Yusef had once again spun out of control. He had no apartment, no wife, and something resembling Damocles' sword dangling over his head.

His mother, now used to such situations, took him in but laid down the law. "She was really mad," recalls Yusef. "She said I was full of shit when I gave her a story of why Jamillah and I broke up. She said, 'I knew you would fuck up.' She told me I'd have to get a job, and she'd be keeping the paycheck. Even a sniff of drugs or any criminal activity would result in me being thrown out."

Yusef's attempts to clean himself up were always halfhearted and doomed to failure. This time was no different. He enrolled in a drug-treatment program and started taking methadone. Gradually, Yusef began attending *juma* services at the mosque. One day he spotted Jamillah and they started talking. It wasn't difficult; the mutual attraction was still strong. They agreed to see each other outside the mosque. A date, which began at a neighborhood restaurant and progressed to a local movie theater and a night at a motel, sealed their continuing interest in each other.

But those positive steps were offset by Yusef's periodic use of alcohol and heroin, and the boosting of commercial merchandise to pay for the spirits and drugs. Caught stealing meat from a supermarket, Yusef found himself back in prison awaiting trial. His petty crime was a small blip on the screen of the Court of Common Pleas judges, who were now seeing considerably more violent crimes on their dockets, and Yusef was quickly given probation and sent to a drug-treatment program. Another halfhearted rehabilitative effort led to another probation violation, and once again shoplifting landed him in a prison cell block.

Yusef's probation officer, a young, progressive white man, took an interest in him. He saw that Edward Anthony was more a perpetual screwup than a real threat to society. There was no doubt Anthony had a problem with drugs and making decisions, but he was likable, wasn't violent or confrontational, and, given the right counseling and treatment, he just might break out of this cycle of self-destructive behavior. The probation officer suggested a somewhat unusual programmatic game plan to Yusef, one that would take him out of state and place him in a long-term intensive treatment program. The alternative was another prison term, and Yusef jumped at the opportunity to participate in something that represented hope rather than failure.

He was taken before a federal judge, who sentenced him to a seven-month term at Lexington Federal Penitentiary in Kentucky, one of the oldest and best treatment programs behind bars for those with addictive diseases. After an arduous eighteen-hour bus ride, a prison official boarded the bus and told the men, "Welcome to Lexington. If you have any drugs on you, you better take them now, because they'll be the last drugs you see for the duration of your time here." That unusual welcome was an apt introduction to what Yusef and the others would face at Lexington.

"Compared to the county jail," says Yusef, "Lexington was certainly an improvement. They really tried to work with you and help you there. You had to be diligent, conscientious, and constantly open to discussing your problems. The goal was to help you change your life. It really was better than anything I had seen in the Philly prisons. One of the more surprising things, for example, was that there weren't really cells, but actual rooms. At first there were three of us in a room, but as you progressed in the program you were rewarded with a room of your own.

"There was a lot of therapy sessions, both one-on-one and group sessions. And there were a lot of activities besides the therapeutic programs, including all sorts of gym activities and sports, and they even took some of us out to visit local schools in a kind of scared-straight program to educate kids about the evils of drugs and crime. Occasionally they'd make us write five-hundred- and six-hundred-word introspective compositions about our lives and hopes for the future.

"Several times I got pissed off at the therapists and group session leaders and said, 'Look, you tell me what's wrong with me. You're the one with the college degrees. You're the damn therapist. Why am I like this? I go through all these damn programs and work to get off drugs, and then when they're over I start right back up again with them. Sometimes before I even get home. Why is that? Why doesn't anything work?'"

Yusef never received a satisfactory answer, but he thrived in the Lexington program, becoming a trusted worker and a willing, good-natured participant in all the institution's scheduled activities. His only difficulties were related to his health. His gastrointestinal problems were always a source of concern, but over the years he had learned to live with a constantly bloated stomach, chronic indigestion, and a diet heavy on roughage. He was also constantly in search of laxatives that would enable something resembling normal and regular bowel movements. The diet study at Holmesburg and the subsequent hemorrhoid surgery had left their mark.

Of more concern, however, was a recurrence of his skin ailment. "My skin started to break out again," says Yusef, "and my hands and feet began to swell up. I said to myself, 'Oh no, not again. Am I always going to be cursed with this stuff?'"

Yusef immediately consulted the prison doctors in the hope of avoiding another catastrophic situation. He informed them of his health history, the prison experiments and their impact, and his more recent month-and-a-half stint in Philadelphia General Hospital. The doctors theorized that he might have come into contact with something at Lexington that had triggered the recurrence and removed him from his job as a painter on the maintenance crew. In addition, he was given several creams and lotions and was allowed to soak his hands and feet in various medicinal solutions whenever he felt it necessary.

The swelling gradually receded to an acceptable level, but Yusef was still hampered in the jobs he could be assigned and none too thrilled with the stigma that came of having to be handled with kid gloves for fear of another recurrence of his bizarre skin malady. He was also becoming resigned to the fact that medical research had given him an array of lifetime disabilities.

After seven months Yusef was released from Lexington. He returned to Philadelphia and was forced to get a room at a Center City YMCA, as his mother had taken in some struggling relatives during his imprisonment. Though his prospects for work and life were far from bright, he did show some newfound resolve and turned down the opportunity to shoot drugs on several occasions. That significant advance, however, was quickly countered

"A Righteous Life"

by several setbacks. It wasn't long before mounting employment and housing reversals threw Yusef into a grinding depression. Forced once again to ask his mother for shelter, he became consumed by the hopelessness of it all.

"I was sleeping on the living room couch," recalls Yusef. "My mother was pressuring me to get a job, and telling me to contribute to the upkeep of the house when not demanding I move out and get a place of my own. I just got so frustrated. I just said fuck it. I started using again."

He was introduced to the Dilaudid and morphine tablets that were now popular in the community, which could be easily dropped in water and the mixture shot up with a syringe. Yusef was back in the swing of things. It was now a new decade, the 1980s, but he was right back where he'd started nearly two decades earlier. He hadn't been home from Lexington a week.

Several arrests followed. All shoplifting charges, one was for swiping meat from a supermarket, another for stealing sweaters from a discount clothing store. There was even one for palming a package of Contact cold medicine from a pharmacy. Short prison stints followed each one.

But then something unusual happened. After Yusef was nabbed on another shoplifting charge, the assistant district attorney argued vigorously that "the defendant in this case hasn't an ounce of rehabilitation in his entire body. This man's record is disgraceful. He's been going back and forth to prison for 20 years. Obviously, he's not going to change with another county sentence. He's just wasting the county's money. This man requires a state sentence."

Prior to the ADA's outburst, Yusef had expected the judge to hand him no more than an eleven-and-a-half- to twenty-three-month sentence, to be served in the county prison system. Shoplifting, in Yusef's experience, had always been ruled a misdemeanor. Persuaded by the ADA's emotional argument, however, the judge now hit Yusef with a stern lecture and a two- to four-year sentence. Though this was only marginally longer than past sentences, its real import was that Yusef would have to serve the time in a state prison.

Yusef was apprehensive about doing a stint in a large state institution; he had grown used to county time. At least he was familiar with the layout and routine in Holmesburg, the House of Correction, and the Detention Center. After numerous arrests and many years in each, he had learned how to survive and stay out of trouble. He got his first taste of the dramatically different world he was about to enter on the one-hour ride to Graterford in western Montgomery County.

"We were riding in the sheriff's van to Graterford State Penitentiary when we hit a bump," Yusef recalls. "It startled me. I woke up from a deep sleep, and when I opened my eyes, all I could see was this big-ass monster of a wall. Damn, that gray thirty-five-foot-high concrete wall went along as far as the eye could see. It was huge and gave me the shivers. I started thinking of the men they had buried behind that wall, the crimes they had committed, and how much time they must be doing. It all scared the hell out of me."

That forbidding introduction to the largest institution in the state system—and one of the largest in the nation—wasn't softened once Yusef got inside. Built something like a massive telephone pole, Graterford has five incredibly long, double-tiered cell blocks. Yusef was amazed. "Looking down those long blocks with all these killers and murderers on them," he says, "scared me to death. That big-ass fuckin' place was mean. If you had a problem with somebody on the block, it would take the guards two days before they could get to you."

Fortunately, Yusef knew a lot of the men serving time there. In and out of prison for twenty years, he ran into men he hadn't seen for some time. Convicted of far more serious offenses than shoplifting, they were doing serious time. Ten- to twenty- and twenty- to forty-year sentences were common. Some men were serving more than one hundred years, and many were doing life for murder. A number of men along the tier recognized Yusef as he was brought onto A block and called out, "Hey, Brother Butch, welcome to Graterford. How you doin', baby?" "Look who they just brought in—it's our old friend Outer Limits."

Locked on a quarantine block for a battery of psychological and educational tests that would determine in which facility he should serve the bulk of his sentence, Yusef had little chance to roam the institution and meet his neighbors, which was fine with him. Graterford was a hard pill to swallow; he was content to hide in his cell.

Thirty days later Yusef was notified that he was being shipped out, was promptly placed on a bus with three dozen other inmates, and was driven to Huntingdon State Penitentiary in central Pennsylvania. Situated in the rural heartland of the state, Huntingdon was known by urban blacks as a "cold stop." Yusef had heard about it from some of the brothers who had served time there and was naturally apprehensive. "Man, that place looked like a damn medieval castle as we drove up to it," he says. "The place was old. So old the guards had to pull a chain outside your cell after you had finished using the toilet. And it seemed all of the guards were white, backwoods country folk. They let the brothers know just where we stood."

A month later Yusef was placed on another bus and driven across the state to Western State Penitentiary in Pittsburgh. This castle-like structure was even older than Huntingdon, with four- and five-tier cell blocks and cells so small that a person could touch both walls by extending his arms. For the third month in a row Yusef remained in quarantine and went through a battery of exams.

His final dose of diesel therapy—the term prisoners used for the seemingly endless bus rides around the commonwealth—took place on another prison vehicle that traveled back across the state and through the rolling hills of Centre County in the vicinity of Penn State University. Its destination, however, was not the leafy, picturesque college town but the nearby state pen. Rockview was built on the side of a mountain, but its ominous appearance was slightly misleading. In fact, it was a fairly progressive institution whose proximity to the university allowed for a rich diversity of educational programs and visitors.

"There was a greater sense of freedom at Rockview," says Yusef. "Trustees could go to the college and take courses, and many of the students from Penn State majoring in psychology and criminal justice came and worked in the prison. That sort of interaction made for a better situation than at most prisons. You didn't feel so isolated. You could still think of yourself as part of society and the outside world."

Though Yusef's relatively short sentence prevented him from participating in some of the longer, more structured programs, especially those outside the walls, he readily availed himself of a number of educational and therapeutic classes. He was assigned to work in the prison's upholstery shop and thereby reacquainted himself with some of the tools and lessons he had learned in his high school shop classes.

As usual, Yusef recognized a number of inmates from his many trips to Holmesburg, and they remembered him. One of them, Big Herb, recalled Yusef from his first trip to the Burg and insisted on addressing him as Outer Limits. "Hey, Outer Limits," he would call out, "you been seeing any UFOs today? You let me know if you see any spacemen from Mars, okay?" Yusef tried to take the good-natured ribbing in stride. He knew the Holmesburg army experiments had severely altered his personality at the time and that he must have appeared one bizarre character. That so many prisoners remembered him as the loony Outer Limits only underscored that realization. His defensiveness about it was assuaged by the fact that he could take part in some lighthearted bullshit sessions about the Holmesburg medical experiments. He wasn't the only one to have suffered physically or to appear strange and delusional; many other individuals and incidents were fodder for discussion, laughter, and sober reflection.

Yusef also reimmersed himself in his religion and eventually assumed the responsible position of assistant imam for the Sunni Muslims at the institution. He taught basic Arabic and *salat* classes and performed *juma* services every Friday with an imam from the free world who came into the institution. He was determined that, this time, his devout behavior in prison would carry over to the streets upon release.

During his year and a half at Rockview, Yusef also struck up a relationship with another woman. Darlene was a short, light-skinned woman in her midtwenties with two young children. Introduced by a mutual friend, Yusef and Darlene quickly developed an interest in one another. They wrote often and had many enjoyable phone conversations, and she made several trips up to the central Pennsylvania state prison to visit him. The relationship proved helpful not only for the support she offered throughout his incarceration, but also in providing a place to call home once he was released.

Set free in the summer of 1983, Yusef first went back to his mother's house. Not surprisingly, the residual ill will between mother and son, exacerbated by cramped sleeping quarters due to additional relatives' living in the house, led to his departure after two weeks. For once, however, his frustration did not lead to drug use. Ever so slowly, Yusef was finally understanding and successfully grappling with his self-destructive addictive behavior. To the shock of many former friends in the neighborhood, Yusef was declining their invitations to party and get high.

This high-water mark of personal resolve, however, was headed for some hurricane-force winds. How could it be otherwise, given Edward "Yusef" Anthony's history? The most serious threat to his newfound sobriety came from a surprising source—his girlfriend's mother.

"When I left my mother's house," says Yusef, "I was desperate for a place to stay. My parole plan was already a bit shaky, and if I'm homeless the parole board would have thrown my ass right back into prison. Darlene said I could stay with her, and we were getting along real well, but she and her kids were living in her parents' house around 33rd and Lehigh. Her father had had a stroke and was always on oxygen. Her mother was on vodka. Lorraine was an alcoholic, and the first day I'm in there she's telling me, 'If you wanna live in this house, you gotta drink with me.' I'm thinking, what the hell did I get myself into? Right away she pours me a big glass of vodka and wants me to sit and drink with her. I don't want to drink it, but I've really got no choice. I need a place to live; otherwise the state is gonna find one for me."

Resigned to making the best of a bad situation, Yusef knew he had to find work. His various health maladies preventing him from accepting the more strenuous conventional employment opportunities, so he decided to become a street vendor selling incense, exotic oils, and soaps. Long hours and a good knowledge of the city enabled him to survive economically and eventually begin selling an eclectic mix of goods, including socks, electric hair curlers, and telephones.

"I was doing good," says Yusef. "I was making money, I wasn't stealing, and I wasn't using drugs."

But his home life was still precarious. Darlene's mother routinely made him go to the state store to buy her liquor, and Darlene contributed to the problem by occasionally dabbling in street drugs. She wanted Yusef to get high with her, stay home and play cards, and go to parties with her. Though he sometimes succumbed to the various temptations the household presented, Yusef had stopped committing crimes. The many years of boosting merchandise from supermarkets and clothing stores in order to earn a buck had ended. It was a significant milestone.

After spending a good part of the 1980s with Darlene and her family, Yusef decided to leave in 1989. As he says of that frustrating time, "I couldn't deal with it anymore. I was living in a house that was presenting me with nothing but temptation. Alcohol and drugs were always around. I had to get out or I would have been sucked right in again."

He moved in with a friend from the mosque and then to his sister Lucille's, who was caring for older brother Will, another Anthony sibling now struggling with serious coronary disease. Yusef started collecting SSI checks from the government, which helped immeasurably, began contributing to the upkeep of the house, and started taking his religion and personal health far more seriously than ever before.

"I tried to pull myself up by my bootstraps and never look back," Yusef recalls of that significant turn in his life. "I decided as best I could I was gonna try and live a righteous life. I got into my religion, went to the mosque regularly, and made sure I performed *salat* five times a day.

"I also decided to try and improve my health. I was so tired of dealing with physical problems. I now had arthritis in my joints and hepatitis C, in addition to all my other medical issues. My back was in bad shape, and I was really limited in what I could do or lift. I was so depressed about my health, but I really wanted to make a healthy comeback, so I started eating right, exercising, doing sit-ups, jogging, and taking all sorts of herbs and supplements from natural health food stores. I followed an alkaloid diet heavy in fiber and ate a lot of roughage to try and help relieve my stomach problems. I hoped it would also have a beneficial effect on the frequency of my skin eruptions. I did the whole nine yards. I thought I'd try something new, 'cause nothing else seemed to work.

"I said the hell with all those doctors I'd been seeing over the years. They weren't doing anything for me. The new ones I was seeing had no idea what I had or how to treat me, and the ones from Holmesburg were vampires and Frankensteins. They told us at the time they were simple cosmetic tests we were getting on, but in reality they were far more than that. Guys got ruined in there, and I was one of them. The less doctors I saw, the better. I really didn't trust them any longer."

By the mid-1990s Yusef was living alone in a small but comfortable efficiency apartment in the Germantown section of Philadelphia, and following a somewhat monastic lifestyle predicated on quiet spirituality and daily physical maintenance. Reading the Koran, exercising, and following a strict diet became the pillars of his existence. After several decades of terrible self-abuse, illicit drugs and crime were no longer part of his life.

"Trying to Get a Little Justice"

It was a warm, pleasant day in late spring 1998 and Yusef was preparing his evening meal. The food preparation ritual was well rehearsed at this point; health and budgetary constraints dictated a diet heavy on fruits, steamed vegetables, and tofu or veggie burgers in place of meat. The six o'clock news was on, and although he was not paying particularly close attention, he was startled to hear the words "medical experiments," "Holmesburg Prison," and "allegations of unethical conduct." He quickly dropped his kitchen utensils and ran to his small black-and-white television. The network anchorman was talking excitedly about a new book that documented the chilling history of medical research carried out at Philadelphia's Holmesburg Prison. Stock film footage of Holmesburg's ominous exterior and antiquated cell blocks rolled across the TV screen as the anchorman described "experiments utilizing dioxin and radioactive isotopes."

16

Yusef was dumbstruck; he said it was like a fifty-five-gallon container of ice water washing over him. "Man, that just opened the door," he recalled. "All these terrible Holmesburg memories came flooding back. It was terrible."

Soon his telephone began to ring, and for days thereafter friends and acquaintances, many of whom he hadn't heard from in years, began to call and ask, "Did you hear the news last night?" "Did you hear what they were saying about us?" "Did you get a copy of the book yet?"

Yusef had mixed feelings about the excitement now stirring among former Holmesburg prisoners. "It was like tearing off a scab, reopening an old wound that had never quite healed," he says. "I didn't want to think about those days again. They were some of the worst times of my life, and I was still dealing with the effects from those experiments. I was never the same after they had gotten ahold of me, but guys were now learning for the first time what had gone down in there. What we were really being exposed to. Guys would be running down the street to talk to me about another TV news show that had featured the book, and passing around newspaper articles on the book and what it said about the experiments. Headlines would say, 'Acres of Skin Documents Experiments on Prison Inmates,' 'Holmesburg Prisoners Were Human Guinea Pigs,' and 'Book Exposes Mistreatment of Prisoners.' For guys who had gone through Holmesburg, the book's revelations and all the media coverage it was getting was a pretty big thing. No one had ever shown any interest in us before. We were always shunned and cast aside. Now we were front-page news and getting national TV coverage. And we were learning for the first time what was really going on in there.

"At first, I wasn't all that crazy about the hype. It wasn't anything I was too crazy about going through again. I had spent the last thirty years trying to forget what happened to me and dealing with all the problems I had come out of there with. But I couldn't avoid it. Seemed like every time I was listening to the radio or watching TV, there'd be some mention of it. I'd wake up one morning and hear Aaron Brown on *Good Morning America* talking about the book and Holmesburg, and later in the day a local news show doing the same thing. The next day would be the same thing. I'd wake up to another local show interviewing the author, and then later that night I'd see the *CBS Evening News* covering the story. It was really something; Dan Rather was talking about stuff I had gone through. And, in between, guys be calling me saying so-and-so from so-and-so newspaper or TV station wanted to interview them and I should tell them what happened to me. But I still didn't want to get involved; the whole thing was just too painful.

"It wasn't long, though, before I finally got a copy of *Acres of Skin*. I started reading, and right away I thought, it's a shame my name ain't in there. I belonged in that book. The guys in there were messed up, but nothing like I was. They tortured me. It took 'em months to fix me up each time I went on one of those tests, and I still ain't right."

Yusef then received a call about a meeting; many of the former Holmesburg test subjects were getting together. The author of the book had been invited and participants would be encouraged to tell their stories, have their questions answered, and explore any legal alternatives they might have. About two dozen former inmates attended that first meeting, including Yusef, who kept a low profile. He listened intently to the commentaries of others but was reticent about sharing his own powerful Holmesburg recollections. The men passed copies of the book around, pointed to various photos and passages that they identified with, and began to open up about their experiences. The names of others not in attendance were mentioned frequently as individuals who were known to have been on the army tests or were victims of painful biopsies. Many pulled up their shirtsleeves and pant legs to show remnants of the experiments, while others exposed their backs and the lasting scars of forty-year-old patch tests. Some spoke in hushed tones, barely audible, almost as though they were ashamed, while others were more strident and clearly appalled by what the city prison system and the University of Pennsylvania had done to them. Yusef could understand both the timidity and the moral outrage.

One former test subject raised his pant leg and displayed an unsightly, discolored leg, then told of the so-called athlete's foot experiment he had been subjected to, in which powder was put on his right foot and then the foot wrapped in a plastic bag for a week, so no air could get to it. The result, he said, was nerve damage and ugly scarring. Another told of three stomach operations because of liquids he was required to drink as part of a Holmesburg diet test. He said, "I'm trying to get a little justice for some of the experiments done on me." Others echoed those comments and talked of "unfair, barbaric" medical practices and mercenary doctors who had left a lot of men and women broken and resentful.

"Man, just listening to that stuff," says Yusef, "made me feel I was right back in jail again. It felt like I hadn't gone anywhere. I was still locked up. Those early meetings were really painful. I knew I was fucked up, and listening to all those other guys talk about their health problems just made me sick and angry. Those prison tests were the damnation of my whole fucking life."

During the summer and fall of 1998 there were many more meetings, and the group's membership grew exponentially. Each successive meeting garnered a couple dozen new attendees. Word was circulating through working-class Philadelphia neighborhoods; something was brewing, and former inmate test subjects were at the center of it. Though there was a smattering of sixty- and seventy-year-old white men present, the vast majority of those in attendance were African American. The burgeoning

189

group took on the name Experimentation Survivors and did numerous media interviews. They also invited supporters to attend their meetings and help them explore strategies and options.

Stefan Presser, legal director of the American Civil Liberties Union of Pennsylvania, was sympathetic and said their case was compelling, but the amount of medical, dental, and psychological testing needed before litigation could proceed would come to "tens, if not hundreds of thousands of dollars."[1] It would be a daunting process financially, legally, and emotionally.

Harold James, a Pennsylvania state representative, was moved by the personal testimonies and talked of holding investigative hearings on the subject. "I think it's a long time coming," said James, of *Acres of Skin* and the former inmates' desire for treatment and compensation.[2]

When contacted by reporters for a response to the book's allegations and the test subjects' meetings, Richard Tannen, senior vice dean in charge of research and academics at the University of Pennsylvania's School of Medicine, said he believed new hearings were unnecessary and that no one had proved that the Holmesburg experiments had caused long-term complications. Dr. Albert M. Kligman issued a statement saying that his research "was in keeping with this nation's standard protocol for conducting scientific investigations at that time."[3]

Over the course of the next few months, the former Holmesburg Prison test subjects participated in more media interviews, held several protests and demonstrations at Philadelphia City Hall and the University of Pennsylvania, met with lawmakers, and acquired an attorney. Things were happening; there was an air of excitement, and anything seemed possible. "Something good may yet happen with this," Yusef started to believe. "We were getting information out to the public. I and the others wanted to make sure the stuff they did to us never happened again. All the attention we were getting made me hopeful. Maybe there'd be some sunshine at the end of all this."

In addition to the goals of remuneration and public education, Yusef was hoping for something personal. "I used to go by this center city clinic that specialized in repairing damaged fingers and hands and thought it would be great if they'd take a look at me. But I knew it would never happen. They didn't take Medicaid cards. It was one of those specialty hospitals that just catered to rich people or people with insurance, and I'd just sit on the bus and think about it when I'd be going by. People would always stare at my hands and sometimes move away from me, thinking I must have some strange disease. Yeah, I started thinking about that hand clinic. Maybe it was possible."

The former test subjects also began speaking to students on college and university campuses. Though nervous about such appearances and apprehensive about showcasing his modest public speaking abilities, Yusef was periodically drafted to enter a college classroom and talk about his experience as an imprisoned human guinea pig. For the high school dropout, ex-criminal, and longtime drug user, it was a traumatic experience.

"It was a really hard thing to do," says Yusef. "I'm basically an introvert, and to stand up in front of a class of students was nerve-wracking. It was especially hard, not only because I had to talk about my own fucked-up life, but I had to tell it to mostly white kids who didn't know about the kind of things I went through. Most of them came up with the best of everything and were now getting a college education and were gonna become lawyers and doctors and professional people. Hell, I never even graduated high school. I was a functional illiterate and probably did more time in prison than they had lived on this earth.

"I'd be so nervous before going into one of those classes, I'd have to take some Valiums to calm my nerves. I don't know if they knew how nervous I was. On a couple of those early visits I know I started crying, and that was really embarrassing. Opening up about my life and those experiments was really difficult. At night I'd end up with nightmares about the experiments. I sure as hell didn't look forward to doing it. To be honest, I always looked for an excuse to get out of going up there."

His early appearances at Temple University in Philadelphia were unsteady, fitful performances that necessitated his being asked a series of questions, such as, "How old were you when you first entered Holmesburg?" "What were you charged with?" "When did you first take notice of the clinical trials at the prison?" He couldn't transition from one subject to another without being prompted; he needed a rigid Q & A format.

Despite his obvious anxiety, however, there were positive signs that the public-speaking gigs wouldn't always be the mountain-sized obstacles they appeared to be at first. Once he got going on a subject, such as his initial prison patch test or the army psychotropic drug test, he seemed to lose his nervousness, and then he gave an illuminating—indeed, a chilling—account of his experience. Students sat spellbound. Some noticeably winced or cringed as Yusef described the strawberry-red pustules that covered his skin,

191

his hands increasing in size until they resembled boxing gloves, or his bizarre transformation in reaction to the army's chemical experiments. Invariably, students would come up to him after his lecture, shake his hand, and thank him for coming to speak to the class. The immediate feedback and genuine expressions of support were cathartic; it was almost better than money.

His appearances at Temple were quickly followed by presentations at Stockton State College in New Jersey and at West Chester State, Holy Family College, and Chestnut Hill College, all in Pennsylvania. But his college speaking tour wasn't limited to the Philadelphia area. Yusef was also invited into the prestigious Ivy League, lecturing at Brown University not once but twice. The flights to Rhode Island were his first in a jet, and the pristine Providence campus was a welcome change of pace from normal Philadelphia haunts. The former drug addict and inveterate shoplifter was now a much appreciated and sought-after spokesman on a very dark subject in American medical history.

Regrettably, the efforts of Yusef and his Holmesburg confederates did not translate into political muscle, legal victories, or financial remuneration. Although the *Acres of Skin* exposé had kicked off a campaign that garnered prominent coverage in such faraway places as Washington (*Seattle Times*), California (*Los Angeles Times*), Texas (*Houston Chronicle*), and New York (*New York Times* and the *Village Voice*), along with international news organizations such as the BBC, not to mention very favorable local media, the campaign was far from a political tour de force. Organizations, whether civic or religious, didn't gravitate to the banner of the Experimentation Survivors. It might have been different if the survivors had been orphans or the mentally retarded or senile, or senior citizens, or any of the other vulnerable groups that were subjected to experimentation in postwar America, but these men were former criminals, and overwhelmingly African American to boot.

Negotiations to reach a settlement between the lawyer for the test subjects and Penn, the City of Philadelphia, and a pharmaceutical company proved disappointing. And although a second attorney hired by the group filed suit for approximately three hundred plaintiffs, the results were equally discouraging. A federal judge ruled that Pennsylvania's discovery rule and strict statute of limitations had required lawsuits to be filed within a narrow two-year window of opportunity from the date when the plaintiffs knew or should have known they had been injured. Even though many of the former test subjects were illiterate or were forced to sign deceptive liability waivers, the judge argued that there had been ample time to learn of their injuries and that suits should have been filed many years earlier. The decision severely crippled their legal options.

Despite the negative turnabout, Yusef and his compatriots continued to press their case wherever and however they could. When informed that a prestigious medical society would be presenting Dr. Kligman with a lifetime achievement award, they were appalled. How, they wondered, could any organization honor someone who so cavalierly used children, senior citizens, and prisoners in unethical medical experiments?

"They got a hell of a nerve," said Yusef of the event's organizers. "Kligman was like Frankenstein. And he never apologized. Those doctors should have been ashamed of themselves for giving an award to somebody who repeatedly took advantage of the poor and the ignorant. Kligman should have been exposed for what he was. It really demonstrated the hypocrisy of the entire medical profession. Once again it was all about money."

Determined not to let the unseemly event go on unnoticed, the former test subjects decided to present the eminent Dr. Kligman with an award of their own. While limousines dropped off tuxedo-attired physicians, former inmates and their supporters established a picket line, voiced their opposition, and tried to give their former tormentor the first annual Joseph Mengele Award. Kligman, the citation proclaimed, had displayed "inhuman actions above and beyond the call of duty" and had participated in the "steady and unrelenting abuse of man." Though the renowned doctor entered the hall through a side door, thereby avoiding a confrontation with protestors, media coverage of the event signaled Dr. Kligman's vulnerability as an honoree and issued a warning to other organizations that might want to honor him: they would be destined for some unwanted publicity and unexpected guests.

Yusef and his fellow activists, however, were not devoid of friends in high places. Pennsylvania state representative Harold James held a legislative hearing in Philadelphia on the impact of the Holmesburg human research program, and Philadelphia city councilman David Cohen, a longtime supporter of disenfranchised groups, organized two council hearings on the subject. Yusef was among a long list of former Holmesburg inmates who presented gripping testimony of their days as test subjects. Many removed their clothing to show council members and media representatives their scars.

Some of the most surprising and compelling testimony presented at those hearings, held on February 22, 1999, and May 7, 2002, came from

A. Bernard Ackerman, one of the world's leading dermatopathologists. As a second-year resident in dermatology at Penn in 1966, Ackerman was an actual witness to what transpired at Holmesburg. "I was told that we were advancing the cause of medicine . . . giving prisoners the opportunity to participate in the advance of science . . . affording them the chance to be technicians and medical assistants upon their release from prison, and offering them the possibility of earning more money than they could in any other institution," said Dr. Ackerman. "In fact, what was purported to be a research institute at Holmesburg . . . was little more than a commercial operation in which Dr. Kligman, the University of Pennsylvania, and possibly others, reaped huge financial dividends." Not once, said Ackerman, "was there a single attempt, in word or deed, on the part of the University of Pennsylvania to oversee what transpired, medically and ethically, at Holmesburg."[4]

The fact that a preeminent physician and researcher was breaking ranks with his medical colleagues and documenting the many unethical lapses that occurred at Holmesburg did not go unnoticed by those in attendance. Both lawmakers and members of the audience knew they were witnessing something highly unusual. As Yusef said afterward, "Man, that doctor really nailed it. He really told the truth."

Ackerman concluded his remarks by stating that Penn had clearly abdicated its "responsibility to the prisoners," as well as to the university's medical "trainees." There was a clear responsibility, said Ackerman, "to set standards, to alert to violations of the Nuremberg Code, and to ensure that the research done under their authority was serious and meaningful. It did nothing of the sort. It had an obligation to us to set standards for informed consent. It did not. It had an obligation to us to mandate that scientific work at Holmesburg was truly scientific. It did not. It had an obligation to us to make a clear distinction between commerce and medicine. It did not."

Despite such forceful testimony and the former inmates' display of scars and lasting infirmities, there would be little in the way of tangible results. Requests for apologies from the perpetrators, medical examinations for those still suffering, and financial remuneration for the victims went unanswered. The Experimentation Survivors had organized, protested, filed a lawsuit, and educated the public about an unconscionable event in the nation's medical history, but they had little to show for it. It was a severe blow for many. "I thought we were doing something positive," says Yusef. "I thought this would be the end of a long, hard road. Things looked so hopeful with the release of the book and the interest in our story, but in the end, nothing. It was a big letdown. It's really a hurtin' thing."

Years earlier, such a dramatic and disappointing turn of events would have caused Yusef to sink into one of his hopeless, self-devouring depressions. Undoubtedly he would have picked up a syringe as a means of escape. Invariably shoplifting and imprisonment would have followed. But Yusef was no longer the weak, stressed-out Brother Butch from the Village in North Philly who was so well known for his heroin addiction, boosting, and bad decisions. Although they had dominated a good portion of his life, drugs, crime, and prison were things of the past. Life's disappointments could no longer be counted on to unhinge the former Edward Anthony.

Yusef Abdul Sadiquu still had his daily trials, however. His medical problems alone were a laundry list of physical and mental maladies that ran, literally, from head to foot. Migraine headaches, neuropathy of the face, a herniated disc in his neck, degenerative rheumatoid arthritis of the spine and joints, hepatitis C, and unending gastrointestinal problems presented hourly challenges. Of course, not all of these maladies were necessarily the result of the prison experiments, nor could all the ailments of the other test subjects always be blamed entirely on those experiments. But most of the men, and many of their family members, attributed many of their health problems—particularly in the African American community—to the tests performed on them. And for good reason. They were treated like lab rats, and no follow-up exams were ever performed to gauge the long-term impact of participating in the clinical trials. Information was withheld from them, and they were occasionally deceived outright. It is only natural that the former test subjects would attribute their physical maladies to the tests.

If these maladies weren't burdensome enough, Yusef was diagnosed as a paranoid schizophrenic. Fortunately, his religion and his wife (he and Jamillah had gotten back together) became lighthouses of guidance and stability. Islam and reuniting with Jamillah provided him with hope, emotional sustenance, and happiness.

Today Yusef is a highly respected member of his community. Goodnatured and always willing to provide a helpful hand despite his physical limitations, he is often seen counseling youngsters in the neighborhood on the value of a good education, establishing a healthy lifestyle, and the dangers of drugs. College students repeatedly express amazement at his story, equanimity, and perseverance.

"I've learned an awful lot over the years," says Yusef. "I no longer blame other people for my shortcomings. I used to put things on other people rather than myself. Now I can deal with my faults and try to do better in the future. I see things more clearly now. It hasn't been easy, and I still have problems, but I no longer contribute to those problems with bad decisions. I try to do the best I can each day."

On August 1, 2006, the Institute of Medicine of the National Academy of Sciences presented a report to federal officials that was widely interpreted by prison reform advocates and members of the media as turning back the clock and reopening prison doors to large-scale medical and pharmaceutical testing. Although the authors of the three-hundred-page report, *Ethical Considerations for Research Involving Prisoners*, claim to have recognized "past abuse in biomedical research in prisons" and the "deep distrust it engendered amongst prisoners," they ultimately conclude that "research affords the potential of great benefit" and will "help policy makers better understand and respond to the myriad health problems faced by prisoners."[1]

Citing the growing AIDS and hepatitis C epidemics in our nation's prisons, confusion over the scope of federal regulations (45 C.F.R. 46, subpart C), and the belief that a prisoner's views "should be taken into account" if he or she "wants to participate in research," proponents of the report argue that implementation of several precautionary measures and procedural safeguards will prevent the medical abuses of the past. Incorporating "enhanced systematic oversight" such as conscientious institutional review boards and increased prisoner representation in decision making, they believe, will provide the transparency needed for inmate test subjects and the public to rest assured that abuse will not occur.

Edward "Yusef" Anthony and I beg to differ. More than forty years of intimate involvement in prisons—both here and abroad—has taught us that true prison reform, in whatever manifestation, is either illusory, ephemeral, or so watered down that it is merely a charade orchestrated by those in power. The history of imprisonment in America is one of good intentions gone awry, bad practices solidified, and hope all but extinguished. Much as they were almost two hundred years ago, prisons today are our concrete and steel repositories for social malefactors—miniature, landlocked Devil's Islands reserved for the worst of us. Most people believe that those interned there well deserve the harsh treatment they receive. Little has changed in these fearsome institutions over the years, except that there are considerably more of them, and those warehoused inside are of a decidedly darker hue.

Proposals trumpeting the benefits of medical research on prisoners should be examined with great skepticism, especially considering the sordid history of such practices and the meager state of healthcare in penal institutions today. As Paul Wright, editor of *Prison Legal News*, has stated regarding the IOM recommendations, "It strikes me as pretty ridiculous to start talking about prisoners getting access to cutting-edge research and medications when they can't even get penicillin and high-blood-pressure pills. I have to imagine there are larger financial motivations here."[2]

Do the 2.3 million Americans locked behind bars—many of whom need treatment in mental facilities, not incarceration—represent a virtual goldmine of raw material for a biomedical industry that is supposedly "facing a shortage of test subjects"? Or are they a federated wholesale department store for valuable body parts? Recent legislation introduced in Missouri and South Carolina has offered prisoners reduced sentences and reprieves from death row if they are willing to give up a key body part such as a kidney or bone marrow. Is the commodification of body parts and human beings something we really want to foster?

This certainly isn't the first time the medical and pharmaceutical professions have taken a utilitarian view of such precious resources. In the aftermath of World War II, the U.S. government put twenty-three Nazi doctors and medical administrators on trial in Nuremberg, Germany, for their role in performing gruesome medical experiments on concentration camp prisoners. After lecturing, haranguing, and executing seven of the defendants and sentencing many others to long prison terms, American jurists crafted ten principles to ensure that members of the medical profession would never again abuse research subjects. The critical first principle not only emphasizes that "the voluntary consent of the human subject is absolutely essential," but stipulates, in addition, that subjects "should be so situated as to be able to exercise free power of choice, without the intervention of any element of force, fraud, deceit, duress, overreaching, or other ulterior form of constraint or coercion." The Nuremberg principles would appear to put prisons off limits as sites for medical experimentation.

Ironically, though many nations did subscribe to the Nuremberg Code, the nation that wrote the code did not. Research physicians in America found the wealth of human material in our orphanages, mental hospitals, and institutions for the indigent too useful to be declared untouchable. Institutionalized populations, especially those behind bars, had great medical value for these researchers.

In fact, an argument can be made that penal institutions that evolved into large-scale pharmaceutical testing factories, such as Holmesburg and Jackson State Prison in southern Michigan, were the northern equivalent of the brutal convict-leasing system so prevalent in the postbellum South. Instead of being held in prison farms like Parchment in Mississippi, and being rented out to private interests to perform backbreaking labor digging canals, clearing swamps, and picking cotton, prisoners in fortress-like institutions in the North were lent out as human guinea pigs to the scientific community. Pfizer, Parke-Davis, Upjohn, SmithKline, and Johnson & Johnson became the contractors, just as white planters and mine owners were in the South. Not until the shocking revelations of the Tuskegee syphilis study in the early 1970s did the American public become aware of the terrible damage done to vulnerable institutionalized populations in the postwar years.

Now, in the early years of the twenty-first century, we are witnessing another concerted effort to regain access to that wealth of testing material inside our nation's burgeoning prison system.

"They may have good intentions," says Yusef Anthony of the IOM report, "but jail is too risky and corrupt a place to have tests on humans. Whatever comes in those places is gonna get outta hand. It's gonna turn into something far worse and more dangerous than they ever expected. The protocols and testing may start off proper, but once the public is no longer watching, it will take a totally different direction. I know what goes on in these prisons. They told us years ago, everything will be all right. All the research is safe, and being done by the best doctors. But look what they did to me and all the other guys. I don't believe them anymore."

Prisons are truly unique institutions. Their design, purpose, and paramilitary operation are not intended to foster transparency, encourage free expression, ensure personal privacy, or instill democratic spirit. And prison walls not only do an excellent job of keeping inmates inside, they do an equally fine job of keeping the public out. Medical research is too important, too potentially dangerous, and too sensitive to be carried out in a closed environment housing mostly poor, illiterate, desperate people. The history of the relationship between medical research and prisons in America is not a very comforting one. Uncomfortable to recall, it would be a travesty to relive.

"The thought of prison experiments coming back," says Yusef, "is pretty frightening. I don't want to see any more young, dope-addicted brothers caught up in that experimental meat grinder. When I was arrested and first went to prison, I knew I was gonna be punished, but I thought that meant being locked up and separated from your family and friends. Hell, I was naïve enough to think they might even help me with my drug and alcohol problems. I can assure you, I never thought I'd end up a human guinea pig for some doctor's experiments. A lot of medical people and corporations made serious money from those tests, but all we ended up with was scars, bad memories, and a life of pain. It was wrong the first time they did that stuff to us. I don't believe they deserve a second shot."

Epilogue

1. The complete story of the Holmesburg Prison medical experiments is covered in Allen M. Hornblum, *Acres of Skin: Human Experiments at Holmesburg Prison* (New York: Routledge, 1999).

2. See Todd L. Savitt, "The Use of Blacks for Medical Experimentation and Demonstration in the Old South," *Journal of Southern History* 48, no. 3 (1982): 331–48.

3. A number of books explore the use of vulnerable people as medical test subjects. Some of the better ones include James H. Jones, *Bad Blood: The Tuskegee Syphilis Experiment* (New York: Free Press, 1981); Eileen Welsome, *The Plutonium Files: America's Secret Medical Experiments in the Cold War* (New York: Random House, 1999); Sheila M. Rothman and David J. Rothman, *The Willowbrook Wars* (Somerset, N.J.: Transaction Publishers, 2005); Jonathan Moreno, *Undue Risk: Secret State Experiments on Humans* (New York: Routledge, 2000); John D. Marks, *The Search for the Manchurian Candidate: The CIA and Mind Control* (New York: W. W. Norton, 1979); Susan E. Lederer, *Subjected to Science: Human Experimentation in America Before the Second World War* (Baltimore: Johns Hopkins University Press, 1997); and M. H. Pappworth, *Human Guinea Pigs: Experimentation on Man* (Boston: Beacon Press, 1966).

CHAPTER 2

1. Thomas J. Gibbons was quoted in several newspaper articles on the murder of Chris Schauer in December 1956.

2. Charles Shaw, "The Jungle: Seven Square Miles That Shame—and Menace—Our City," *Philadelphia Sunday Bulletin*, February 3, 1957, News and Views section, 1.

3. Ibid.

4. Shaw's article ignited a flood of commentary in the print media. The articles and letters used for this chapter include Harriett Smith, "Neighbors Disown North Phila. 'Jungle,'" *Philadelphia Evening Bulletin*, February 17, 1957; "The Other Side of 'the Jungle'" (editorial), *Catholic Standard and Times*, February 22, 1957; "Placing the Blame" (unsigned letter), *Philadelphia Evening Bulletin*, February 7, 1957; Alexander Powals, "Grand Exodus Seen," *Philadelphia Evening Bulletin*, February 7, 1957; and C. W. Griffith, "Merely to Shock," *Philadelphia Evening Bulletin*, February 7, 1957.

5. Robert Dreyer, "Boundaries Questioned," *Philadelphia Evening Bulletin*, February 7, 1957.

6. Henry Thomas Dolan, "Jungle Called Degrading Term," ibid., September 12, 1964.

7. Foster Dunlap, "Plain Truth About the Jungle," ibid., February 7, 1957.

8. Kos Spmonski, "Mayor Calls Area the Worst in the City," ibid., May 20, 1961.

9. "2–4 Shoots 2–8 at Corner of 2–7," ibid., April 15, 1964.

10. A Corner Boy, "Why I Got in the Corner," *Dig This Now*, November 12, 1969.

CHAPTER 3

1. Based across town in another section of North Philadelphia known as Kensington, the K & A Gang consisted predominantly of blue-collar Irish burglars who revolutionized the art of burglary from the 1950s to the 1970s. Working in four-man teams and invading several homes per night from Maine to Florida, they managed to earn themselves a handsome living while driving both law enforcement and private homeowners to distraction. The most comprehensive account of the gang is Allen

NOTES

M. Hornblum, *Confessions of a Second Story Man: Junior Kripplebauer and the K & A Gang* (Fort Lee, N.J.: Barricade Books, 2006).

2. Both aspects of Holmesburg's sordid history as well as several others can be found in Hornblum, *Acres of Skin*. Information on the floggings and the Klondike can also be obtained from "Prisoners Beaten on Sorber's Orders," *Philadelphia Bulletin*, February 26, 1929, and "Earle Bares Secret Device for Holmesburg Torture," *Philadelphia Bulletin*, August 31, 1938.

CHAPTER 4

1. Tom Shouler, interview by author, June 14, 1997.
2. Scott Willson, interview by author, December 12, 1994.
3. Priscilla Becroft, interview by author, November 24, 1994.
4. See Hornblum, *Acres of Skin*, 75–118.
5. See Elizabeth W. Etheridge, *The Butterfly Caste: A Social History of Pellagra in the South* (Westport, Conn.: Greenwood Publishing, 1972), 7.
6. L. L. Stanley, "An Analysis of One Thousand Testicular Substance Implantations," *Endocrinology* 6 (1922): 787.
7. "Felons Gather for Test," *New York Times*, March 26, 1934, 24.
8. Hornblum, *Acres of Skin*, 80–84.
9. *Life* magazine, June 4, 1945, 43.
10. David J. Rothman, *Strangers at the Bedside: A History of How Law and Bioethics Transformed Medical Decision Making* (New York: Basic Books, 1991), 51.

11. Walter Rugaber, "Prison Drug and Plasma Projects Leave Fatal Trail," *New York Times*, July 29, 1969, 1.
12. Hornblum, *Acres of Skin*, 75–118.
13. Ibid., 93.
14. Chester M. Southam, interview by author, June 28, 1996.
15. Quoted in Herman Beerman and Gerald S. Lazerus, *The Tradition of Excellence: Dermatology at the University of Pennsylvania, 1870–1985* (Philadelphia: University of Pennsylvania Press, 1986), 132.
16. Quoted in Hornblum, *Acres of Skin*, 37.
17. Ibid., 35.
18. Ibid., 40.
19. See *Acres of Skin* for a fairly detailed accounting of Dr. Kligman's Holmesburg research. Though it is quite possible that numerous other experiments not known to me did take place there, a good many others, from the Phase I pharmaceutical studies to the chemical warfare experiments, the dioxin experiments, and the radioactive isotope experiments, are comprehensively described in the book.

CHAPTER 5

1. It was not terribly unusual for a guard, social worker, or teacher in the Philadelphia prison system to be approached by an obviously stressed, slightly built prisoner requesting help after being pressured for sex by other members of the inmate population. Many young, newly admitted inmates told me of their concerns about being solicited for sex by older prisoners or targeted for attack by prison gangs. Unfortunately, apart from requesting administrative segregation and being locked down twenty-four hours a day, there was little that could be done for these prison novices. As Edward Anthony has said, if you were young, inexperienced in the prison culture, and without friends "to watch your back," you were in serious trouble.

Notes

2. Numerous newspaper articles dealt with the prison rape issue. See, for example, William B. Collins, "Lab Testing Program Tied to Prison Sex Corruptions" *Philadelphia Inquirer,* September 12, 1968, 1.

3. Alan Davis, "Sexual Assaults in the Philadelphia Prison System and the Sheriff's Vans," December 1968.

CHAPTER 6

1. The term is taken from the best-selling book and movie of the same name, which explored the brainwashing of soldiers for political purposes. The best account of the military's and CIA's attempt to discover potent chemical warfare agents is John Marks's *Search for the Manchurian Candidate.*

2. James S. Ketchum, David Kitzes, and Herbert Copelan, "EA 3167: Effects in Man," Edgewood Arsenal, Aberdeen Proving Grounds, Maryland, 21010, January 1975.

3. Hornblum, *Acres of Skin,* provides a detailed account of Dr. Kligman's and Holmesburg's reputation for hosting investigational research on humans. Dozens of pharmaceutical companies, and numerous other private- and public-sector entities, entered into business relations with Dr. Kligman. A number of these relationships are explored in *Acres of Skin,* including those with R. J. Reynolds, Dow Chemical, and the U.S. Army.

4. Report of the Inspector General, Department of the U.S. Army, 1975.

5. Ibid., 158.

6. Lawrence Byrne, interview by author, December 7, 1994.

7. James S. Ketchum, interview by author, February 15, 1995.

CHAPTER 7

1. While many men have learned to read and realize their potential (and become politically conscious) while incarcerated, *The Autobiography of Malcolm X,* as told to Alex Haley (1965), remains the classic work on the subject.

2. See Claude Andrew Clegg, *An Original Man: The Life and Times of Elijah Muhammad* (New York: St. Martin's Press, 1997), 106.

3. Ibid., chapter 3, "The Knowledge of Self and Others," presents one of the better accounts of the Nation of Islam's religious philosophy.

4. I spent the 1970s working in the Philadelphia prison system and saw firsthand the paramilitary type of organization the Nation of Islam had established in the jails. Special handshakes, verbal greetings, hierarchical rank, and marching en masse were all part of the Muslim movement. Inmates who were thought to have made blasphemous comments regarding the NOI or its leader Elijah Muhammad were normally verbally rebuked and occasionally physically abused in some manner.

5. Sean Patrick Griffin, *Black Brothers, Inc.: The Violent Rise and Fall of the Philadelphia Black Mafia* (Preston, UK: Milo Books, 2005), provides a detailed account of the individuals, methods, and violent incidents that made Temple No. 12 particularly notorious.

CHAPTER 16

1. Herbert Lowe, "Used in Lab Tests, Ex-Inmates at Holmesburg Call for Justice," *Philadelphia Inquirer,* September 29, 1998, City and Regional Section, 1.

2. Ibid.

3. Ibid.

4. A. Bernard Ackerman, Testimony before the Philadelphia City Council, May 7, 2002.

EPILOGUE

1. National Academy of Sciences, Institute of Medicine, *Ethical Considerations for Research Involving Prisoners,* July 12, 2006, xii.
2. Quoted in Ian Urbina, "Panel Suggests Using Inmates in Drug Trials," *New York Times,* August 7, 2006, 1.

Notes

Institute of Medicine, 197
Isla, 167–68

Jack, Beau, 15
Jaffa, 173, 176
James, Harold, 190
Jeff's Grocery Store, 16, 35
Jehovah's Witnesses, 145
Jemillah, 168, 172–73, 175–77
Jerry, 29
Jim Yellow, 121
John's Bargain Store, 16
Johnson & Johnson, 2, 45, 55, 112, 199
Joseph Mengele Award, 193
"the jungle," 9

K&A Gang, 36
Kelly, Joseph, 151
Kligman, Albert Montgomery, 52–53, 72, 190, 193
Klondike, 38
Koran, 144–45

Laura, 30–35, 79, 92, 111–13, 115–16
Leopold & Loeb, 50
Lewis, Joe, 15
Lexington Federal Penitentiary, 178
Libbey's Clothing Store, 16
Life magazine, 49
Lindenbaum, Dr., 34
Little Dusty, 122
Little Georgia, 14
Los Angeles Times, 192

Malcolm X (Little), 81
Mama Too Tight, 122
Manhattan, 25
Manhattan General Hospital, 133–34
Masjid Muhajadeen, 156
Mason, John, 154–55
McIntyre Elementary School, 13
Morgan, Lee, 28
Moyamensing Prison, 37–38
Muhammad, Fard, 82, 84, 139
Mustafa, Khalil Abdul, 139–42, 145

Nation of Islam (NOI), 81–82, 85
National Jewish Hospital (Denver), 49
New York Times, 192
Norfolk Prison (Ma.), 81
Nuremberg Code, 50, 52, 194, 198

Olden, George, 123–25, 127
"Outer Limits," 70, 76, 117, 181–82
Overstreet, Lester, 139

Parchment Prison Farm (Miss.), 199
Park Movie Theater, 16, 30
Parke-Davis, 199
Peas, Vincent, 146
Pellagra, 46–47
Penn Fruit, 36
Penn Packing, 114
Penn State University, 182
Pfizer, 199
Philadelphia General Hospital, 91, 101, 112, 162, 179
Presser, Stefan, 190
Prison Legal News, 188

Rather, Dan, 188
Riker's Island, 126
Robins Book Store, 144
Rock & Roll Bar, 16
Rockview State Penitentiary, 182
Rodgers, A. J., 79
Rothman, David, 50

Sadiquu, Yusef Abdul, 195
Schley, Clayton, 15
Schley, Julia, 12
Schmidt, Mike, 49
Seattle Times, 192
Showler, Tom, 43
Sloan-Kettering Institute, 51
SmithKline, 199
Southam, Chester M., 51
Spector, Arlen, 64
Stanley, L. L., 48
Statesville Prison, 49–50
Staton, Dakota, 81
Stennett, Jerome, 81
Stevenson, Gov. Adlai, 49
Stockton State College, 192
Stout, Juanita Kidd, 139
Strawberry Mansion, 12–13

Tannen, Richard, 190
Tanya, 108, 119
Taylor, Leroy, 152–53
Temple University, 191
Tenderloin, 11, 18
Thomas Edison High School, 35, 102

207